Fracture Sonography

Ole Ackermann

Editor

Fracture Sonography

A Comprehensive Clinical Guide

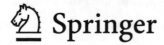 Springer

Editor
Ole Ackermann
Department of Orthopedic Surgery
Ruhr-University Bochum
Bochum
Germany

Based on the translation from the German language edition: Fraktursonografie by Ole Ackermann,
Copyright © Springer-Verlag GmbH Deutschland 2019. All Rights Reserved

ISBN 978-3-030-63841-2   ISBN 978-3-030-63839-9   (eBook)
https://doi.org/10.1007/978-3-030-63839-9

This Springer imprint is published by the registered company Springer Nature Switzerland AG
The registered company address is: Gewerbestrasse 11, 6330 Cham, Switzerland

Foreword

Ever so often you are being asked about progress in your field of expertise, and it is not always easy to point out scientific or clinical progress while you are in the midst of things and working at the bedside. As a consequence, one then tends to believe that procedures and diagnostic tools, especially in our hard-tissue field of orthopedics and skeletal trauma, have developed rather slowly over the last century and that we have done the things we do for decades with only minor improvements, most likely on a technical note.

However, if you step back a little bit and take a broader perspective, you will rather quickly see that the notion above is not the slightest bit true, and that there has been enormous progress on a steadily upward-pointing line for the past century with ever so often some quantum leaps that may not reveal themselves as such at first sight.

To me as an orthopedic surgeon having specialized exclusively in the small sub- or as I like to say "superspecialty" of pediatric musculoskeletal trauma for almost 20 years now, these so-called quantum leaps include for example the advent of elastic stable intramedullary nailing of long-bone fractures inaugurated by METAIZEAU in the 1980s and, in our related field of pediatric orthopedics, the implementation of screening for the dysplastic hip by ultrasound on the base of the achievements by GRAF in the early 1990s.

You can see where this is leading by now, I am sure…

Fracture sonography has been around for a while now; you can trace its beginnings to the publications of LEITGEB in the late 1980s and, with the development of the technique towards higher resolution, the groundbreaking clinical work of our esteemed author, Ole ACKERMANN and others, who analyzed the potential of fracture sonography at different skeletal sites in children and its sensitivity and specificity compared to conventional radiology starting with publications in 2006 and counting.

Within the past decade and based on this work the method has become increasingly popular, also due to the fact that Ole ACKERMANN is a tireless educator for this cause and has established—while continuing his clinical work with patients—a fine curriculum of presence and online coursework which accompanies the wealth of publications in various high-ranking journals as well as the editing of several textbooks.

We are now standing at an exciting new crossroads, and the publication of this new textbook on fracture sonography in children in the English language could not be more timely. Very soon, fracture sonography in children will be standard of care in all emergency rooms specializing in the treatment of children, and it is safe to say that history will repeat itself when comparing the implementation of this diagnostic tool to mandatory hip screening for the early detection of hip dysplasia by ultrasound 20 years earlier.

Finally, it may be added that this progress will literally and figuratively save lives by keeping children away from the unnecessary application of diagnostic radiation, not only at the time of injury but also during follow-up of these fractures.

It has been an honor and an easy task for me to write this short foreword. I am thrilled to see what will happen in the near future in our field with this method, as not only resolution will increase but also 3D-imaging will be possible on a regular basis, which will further add to the dissemination of this great diagnostic tool.

Enjoy reading and "use the force"!

Dirk Sommerfeldt
Altonaer Kinderkrankenhaus
Bleickenallee
Hamburg
Germany

Foreword

Musculoskeletal sonography has expanded immensely over the past two decades, progressing from the radiology suite to the bedside in the hands of clinical providers. Evidence supporting the use of musculoskeletal sonography for diagnosis and management of orthopedic injuries by non-radiologists, with focused training, is available for a large number of applications. Clinicians at the point-of-care, including emergency medicine, orthopedic surgery, sports medicine, trauma surgery, and rehabilitation medicine providers, are using musculoskeletal sonography to improve the care of their patients with orthopedic injuries.

Point-of-care ultrasound can be incorporated into the physical examination at the bedside and applied for almost any musculoskeletal injury. It has been shown to be best for the diagnosis of long bone fractures and detecting fractures as small as 1 mm. However, with techniques including use of a water bath, identification of associated swelling, effusions, or fat pads, and improving ultrasound technology, pathology of the small bones and joints may be accessible by sonography as well. Once a fracture is diagnosed, reduction can be performed with ultrasound guidance, ensuring the best possible re-alignment in all dimensions. In addition, sonography is excellent for diagnosis of joint effusions and dislocations and can assist with procedural arthrocentesis and confirming proper joint relocations.

While sonography is an operator-dependent modality, there is accumulating data that novice sonologists with focused training can accurately diagnose fractures in pediatric patients for a variety of bones. Clinicians performing musculoskeletal ultrasound on children, however, must be able to recognize the normal physes and skull sutures present in a growing child to avoid errors in diagnosis. Importantly, scanning the contralateral normal side for comparison is very useful when unsure if pathology or normal anatomy is present in an area of injury.

Musculoskeletal sonography has many benefits for all populations, but it is especially advantageous in the pediatric population. First of all, sonography does not involve ionizing radiation. Although the radiation from a series of X-rays is low, radiation doses are cumulative for children, and minimizing radiation exposure is always a priority. With up to 80% of obtained radiographs in children negative for fracture, there is a need for an alternative, reliable method to diagnose fractures and reduce the number of X-rays performed. In addition, as sonography can be performed at the bedside, there is no need to transport the child for imaging. Although providers may be hesitant to perform musculoskeletal sonography on an area of injury, children tolerate ultrasound very well when copious gel is applied to the probe, the base of the scanning hand is rested on an uninjured area, the amount of pressure on the injured area is minimized, and the child is allowed to remain in a position of comfort, often in a parent's lap.

In areas with access to radiography, point-of-care ultrasound may facilitate diagnosis and management of orthopedic injuries, thereby decreasing emergency department or clinic length of stay, decreasing overcrowding in medical settings, and decreasing healthcare costs. In austere environments without easy access to radiography, musculoskeletal sonography may be especially valuable. It is estimated that two-thirds of the world's population does not have access to diagnostic imaging. With ultrasound machines becoming more portable, even handheld, with better technology, ultrasound is a logical solution to this lack of diagnostic imaging, especially in resource-limited areas where trauma is a major cause of morbidity and mortality.

This is an exciting time for the growing field of musculoskeletal sonography, with evidence mounting that clinicians with focused training can accurately perform and integrate ultrasound for the benefit of their patients. Dr. Ackermann and his colleagues have done an outstanding job presenting the large variety of musculoskeletal fracture applications and their evidence base. With increased education and resources, including this specialized textbook on Fracture Sonography, clinicians will have access to the high-quality information needed to diagnose and treat their patients around the globe, improving patient management at the point of care.

Joni E. Rabiner
Department of Emergency Medicine
Division of Pediatric Emergency Medicine
New York-Presbyterian Morgan Stanley Children's Hospital
Columbia University Medical Center
New York, NY, USA

Preface

Why fracture sonography? There is a simple and adequate technique with X-ray diagnostics. Anyone dealing with this area will come to this question sooner or later; but also with the answers, each of which alone justified scientific research on the subject.

ALARA

Despite the comparatively low radiation exposure to extremities, we follow the international agreement of the ALARA principle (as low as reasonable achievable). If we can save ionizing radiation with the same level of safety and efficiency, this is a sensible application, especially for patients in growth who have a 5-fold higher radiation sensitivity.

Faster and Smoother

Diagnostics using ultrasound can significantly speed up treatment. Only a single doctor–patient contact is necessary and the time-consuming wait for the X-ray findings is eliminated. With children in particular, there is no need to separate them from their parents and the examination in a dark X-ray room is not necessary. The ultrasound examination in gentle posture and minimal positioning measures as well as the cooling gel is less painful.

Bedside Potential

Ultrasound diagnostics is possible with modern, mobile devices on site (e.g., at sporting events) without radiation protection measures, where radiological diagnostics would require considerable effort (shielded truck). In many cases, an initial assessment is possible in order to ensure optimal continued supply. For certain indications (wrist, excluded elbow and upper arm fractures), the final diagnosis can even be carried out on site.

Further advantages of the technology are the lower costs since suitable devices are available across the board, the possible side comparison of a finding without increased radiation exposure, as well as the possibility of dynamic examination, which allows a stability assessment for fractures.

Of course, there are also disadvantages that should not be neglected. Since this is a new technique, the examiner must first get used to the different display (surface vs. summation image in X-ray), new indications, and specific limitations and dangers. Fracture sonography cannot be used ubiquitously, but only when there is scientific evidence for safe use. This means that the use of ultrasound for diagnostics must be proven separately for each location and each lesion. Furthermore, the use of the method requires specialized training, which currently has to be acquired actively and is not learned on the side. This temporarily means increased stress when ultrasound and X-ray are used in parallel.

A frequently raised objection is the dependency of sonography on the examiner, which as a dynamic examination cannot be adequately documented with static images. In the meantime, we have proven that with correct documentation, a clear review analogous to the X-ray findings is possible. As with the X-ray image, training of the findings is also possible using the ultrasound images.

If the literature of the past years is summarized, the picture of a modern, fast, inexpensive, and safe technology arises, which will expand its spectrum in the coming years. In this book, we have compiled the current state of the evidence.

There are many reports and descriptions of sonographic techniques to visualize fractures, but not all are effective. We chose the methods in this book based on whether they

– can effectively avoid X-ray exposure (e.g., as a reliable exclusion diagnosis)
– provide additional information (e.g., by better measuring the axis deviation)
– are better or equivalent to radiological diagnostics
– make the examination faster and less stressful with the same level of safety
– can be used by a specialist in daily clinical practice

We see the development towards the new techniques. The next few years will certainly show further indications for fracture sonography.

The method must be tested at every location and every fracture entity in order to ensure safe use. For research on the meaningful use of technology, apart from the use in areas or situations with limited resources, there are always three questions to be answered:

(a) Can fracture sonography exclude a fracture with sufficient certainty (and thereby avoid X-rays)?
(b) Does fracture ultrasound provide enough information for safe therapy in the event of a fracture detection (and thereby save X-rays)?
(c) Does fracture sonography provide additional information relevant to therapy that cannot be obtained with less effort?

If at least one of these three questions can be answered positively, it makes sense to use the method in daily routine; if this is not the case, the efficient use of fracture sonography should be critically examined.

Much remains to be done.

Bochum, Germany   Ole Ackermann

Contents

Part I

Introduction

Device Requirements

Ole Ackermann

The equipment requirements for using fracture sonography are low. Only an ultrasound device with a linear transducer is necessary for the examination itself. All transducers from 3.5 to 16 MHz and more are suitable for the examination so that almost all currently used devices can be used for the examination.

Wider transducers offer an advantage when examining long limb bones, narrow ones when imaging small bones.

The possibility of documentation, if possible in digital form, must be available. A buffer of several seconds (CINE) is very helpful and recommended to be able to document the most impressive finding. Since the extremity is held with one hand and the transducer with the other, exact freezing of the optimal image is difficult and only possible with a foot switch.

A preset for bone sonography often does not exist; here the settings for the surface examination have proven themselves.

Ultimately, the possibility of an X-ray examination must be available. Fracture sonography will not replace radiological diagnostics in the foreseeable future and is only useful for certain indications. In addition, an X-ray check must be carried out in the event of doubtful findings. Although this does not always show additional information, it is still the gold standard for many indications.

1.1 Personal Requirements

In addition to the technical requirements described above, the examiner who wants to use fracture sonography independently should have basic skills.

1.1.1 Competence in Ultrasound

Of course, the physical and technical basics of ultrasound technology, device operation, and troubleshooting must be mastered. According to the authors, extensive experience in other areas of ultrasound diagnostics is not absolutely necessary, since the presentation differs fundamentally. In soft tissue sonography, organs are imaged three-dimensionally, in bone sonography essentially two-dimensionally, because for technical reasons no structures can be displayed behind the cortex. The depth as a third dimension is of course available (e.g., when measuring a cortical level), but of minor importance compared to soft tissue sonography.

In this respect, an examiner with little experience in soft tissue imaging can use fracture sonography sufficiently. However, since other questions often arise in clinical practice, e.g., the hematoma or effusion test, a sound education is also useful and recommended in these adjacent areas.

1.1.2 Experience in X-ray Diagnostics

Fracture sonography is not a comprehensive and exclusive diagnosis, it is always to be seen as a supplement and in conjunction with X-ray diagnosis. X-rays have so far been the gold standard and will remain so for many years in most indications, so that the examiner must have access to them at all times. Even though many X-ray images can be saved with the help of sonography, the exclusive use of ultrasound for fracture diagnostics is currently neither sensible nor medically justifiable.

1.1.3 Experience in Fracture Treatment

The interpretation of the findings requires therapeutic competence. As with any diagnostic measure, basic knowledge of the therapy options should be available. This is particularly true for fracture sonography in order to be able to correctly classify the consequences of the findings. For example, it is important to know the dangers of treating child elbow fractures in order to consistently address uncertainties. On the other hand, due to the high correction

O. Ackermann (✉)
Department of Orthopedic Surgery, Ruhr-University Bochum, Bochum, Germany

O. Ackermann (ed.), *Fracture Sonography*, https://doi.org/10.1007/978-3-030-63839-9_1

potential, every minimal lesion on the child's wrist does not have to be extensively clarified if simple and safe therapy is available.

The goal is always to achieve complete diagnostics with minimal effort, which allows adequate therapy.

1.1.4   Training in Fracture Sonography

In order to achieve the necessary reliability in diagnostics, specialized training in fracture sonography is useful. It has already been described above that the display differs from the usual soft tissue imaging. But the fundamental differences to the X-ray image should not be underestimated either. The limited display of each individual image (six ultrasound images are required on the wrist, radiologically only two), the need for precise documentation (the bone shown cannot be determined with certainty later on in the image morphologically) and the pure surface display are difficult for the examiner trained with X-ray diagnostics to get used to. The limits of the display and the special indications for supplementary X-ray diagnostics also require a differentiated examination of the topic.

Training as part of a course therefore makes sense. The following areas must be covered:

1.1.4.1 Theoretical and Scientific Foundations

It must be clear what evidence exists for individual indications and whether comparative studies are available.

1.1.4.2 Indications

Fracture sonography cannot be used universally for all bony lesions. The indications must be clearly stated.

1.1.4.3 Practical Application of the Technology

The clinical practical application in the specific examination courses must be demonstrated and practiced by all participants themselves. Ideally, the examination can be reproduced completely independently. The various cutting planes must be represented reliably and strategies for error correction must be learned.

1.1.4.4 Detect a Fracture

It is important that a course teaches you to recognize a fracture. To do this, the morphological characteristics, sources of error, and standard variants must be discussed. The ability to detect a fracture can be checked using phantoms with normal and pathological findings.

1.1.4.5 Training of Image Diagnosis and Review of Documentation

As with all imaging methods, the correct diagnosis depends above all on the experience of the diagnosis, i.e., the number of images processed so far. This can be trained easily and realistically with computer programs by presenting and practicing a variety of mixed, normal, and pathological findings. At the same time, this procedure trains the review of examinations, as happens in the X-ray discussion. The detection rate can be documented by means of suitable applications and a sufficient ability can thus be demonstrated.

1.2   Radiographs

Fracture sonography is often seen as a method to make X-ray diagnostics superfluous. This is not the case. Fracture sonography can replace X-rays for certain indications, but overall it complements this method and does not replace it.

All currently active doctors have been trained in X-ray diagnostics as the standard procedure for bony lesions and accordingly we trust this technology as the gold standard. This also means that if in doubt, we can fall back on this technology, with which we work safely and reliably everyday.

With all uncertainties in the diagnosis, the additional X-ray examination is always permitted. We assume that additional information only arises in a few cases; for therapy, however, it is necessary that the examiner trusts his own diagnosis. Therefore, especially in the beginning, there is no shame and no failure to take an additional X-ray.

Each examiner will develop their own approach and preferences over time, but everyone will be able to save a lot of X-rays and time with fracture sonography.

Documentation and Artifacts

Christian Schamberger and Ole Ackermann

2.1 Phenomena and Artefacts

Every user who uses B-image sonography for diagnostic purposes should be aware of the relevant phenomena and artefacts that occur during the ultrasound examination in order to be able to reliably assess the sonographic image and avoid incorrect interpretation.

2.1.1 Phenomena

The v of reflex reversal
  The phenomenon of the changing reflex
  The phenomenon of the pseudo usur

2.1.2 Artefacts

Repeating artefact
  Coupling artefact
  Arc artefact
  Posterior acoustic enhancement
  Acoustic shadowing

2.2 Phenomena

Phenomena are special findings in an ultrasound image that have a real reference in the object.

2.2.1 Phenomenon of Reflex Reversal

The phenomenon of reflex reversal occurs when sound waves are not perpendicular reflected back to the transducer when they hit a structure or when the sound waves hit a structure not straight perpendicular. For example, you can see a change in the echogenicity in the area of the insertion of the Achilles tendon at the calcaneus. The echogenicity typically changes from high echogenic (white), where tendon fibres aligned parallel to the ultrasound transducer to low echogenic (dark) when the alignment of the tendon fibres changes when they are fixed to the bone (Fig. 2.1a and b).

Another example is the long head of the biceps tendon in the intertubercular groove in the ventral transverse section plane or the coracoacromial section plane. Depending on the orientation of the transducer, the tendon can be shown either with high echogenicity (white) or low echogenicity (dark, similar to findings in case of a rupture, where the groove is empty) (Fig. 2.2).

2.2.2 The Phenomenon of the Changing Reflex

The phenomenon of the changing reflex is based physically on the same principle as the phenomenon of reflex reversal, but it occurs repeatedly. The sound waves are not all reflected back perpendicular to the transducer, but sent back at different angles or the transducer received the ultrasound waves in different directions due to a wavy tendon shape, i.e., in case of a relaxed patella tendon (Fig. 2.3).

2.2.3 The Phenomenon of Pseudo-usur

If the sound waves strike an object perpendicularly at a convex interface (e.g. capitulum humeri), the convexity at the edge causes sound cancellation of the underlying structure (Fig. 2.4a). In case of a pseudo-usur the parts that are not visible

C. Schamberger
Universitätsklinikum Mannheim, Orthopädisch-Unfallchirurgisches Zentrum, Mannheim, Germany

O. Ackermann (✉)
Department of Orthopedic Surgery, Ruhr-University Bochum, Bochum, Germany

© Springer Nature Switzerland AG 2021
O. Ackermann (ed.), *Fracture Sonography*, https://doi.org/10.1007/978-3-030-63839-9_2

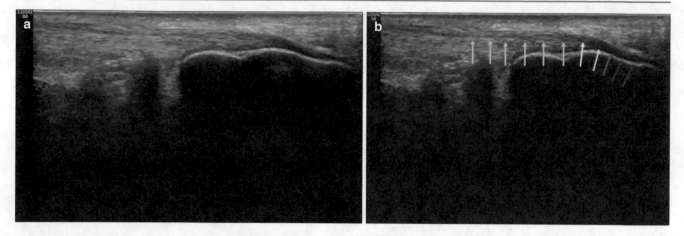

Fig. 2.1 Attachment of the Achilles tendon to the calcaneus, posterior longitudinal section (©Ackermann and Eckert 2015; Courtesy of off label media)

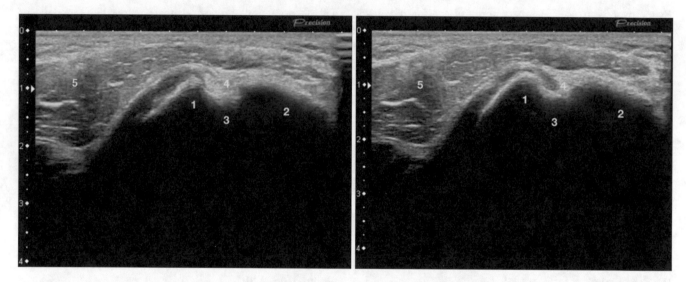

Fig. 2.2 Long biceps tendon in anterior transverse section—orthograde (left) and oblique (right). 1 = Tuberculum minus, 2 = Tuberculum majus, 3 = Sulcus bicipitis, 4 = long biceps tendon, 5 = M. Deltoideus. (©Ackermann and Eckert 2015; Courtesy of off label media)

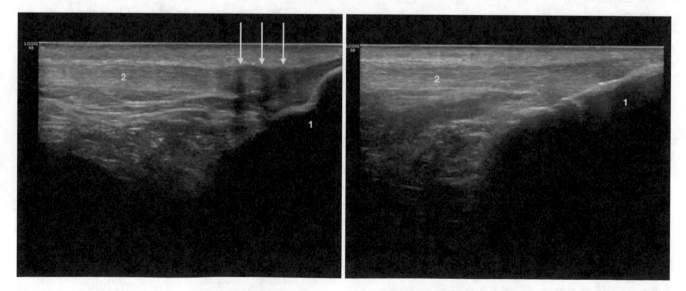

Fig. 2.3 Patellar tendon in a relaxed state with passive hyperextension of the knee joint (left) and tensed state (right) in the insertion area at the tibial tuberosity in an anterior longitudinal section. The arrows mark the wandering reflex. 1 = Tuberositas tibiae, 2 = Patella tendon. (©Ackermann and Eckert 2015; Courtesy of off label media)

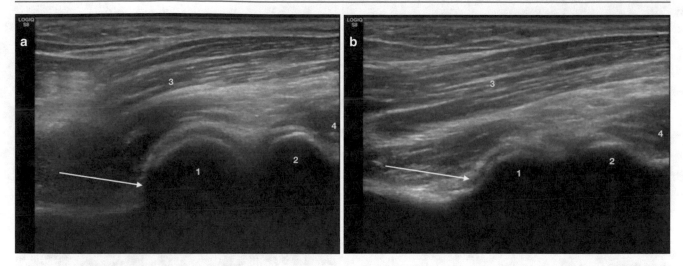

Fig. 2.4 1 = Capitulum humeri, 2 = Radial head, 3 = M. bracioradialis, 4 = M. supinator. White arrow: Pseudo-Usur, when the probe is tilted (Fig. 2.5) the corticalis is visualised. (©Ackermann and Eckert 2015; Courtesy of off label media)

can be shown by simply tilting the transducer. Now the sound waves hit the convex object in the corrected perpendicular direction, the underlying structure can now be displayed and evaluated. This phenomenon is called pseudo-usur (Fig. 2.4b). If the underlying tissue cannot be visualized despite correction of the transducer and there is still an interruption in the bony cortex, it is not a pseudo-usur but a fractura vera.

2.3   Artefacts

In contrast to the phenomena, artefacts are so-called artificial products to which no anatomical structure can be assigned to.

2.3.1   Repetition Artefact

A repetition artefact or repetition echo occurs when the emitted ultrasonic waves are reflected several times at two parallel interfaces (Fig. 2.5). The sound waves cannot return directly to the transducer. Since they now reach the transducer again at different times, an artificial echo is created on the ultrasound image, which is behind the actual echo due to the different time. This artefact can occur, i.e. when using ultrasound gel pads.

2.3.2   Coupling Artefact

A coupling artefact occurs if there is air between the transducer and the skin. This is often found, i.e. in the shoulder examination using the lateral longitudinal section plane when imaging the supraspinatus tendon (Fig. 2.6), in the sec-

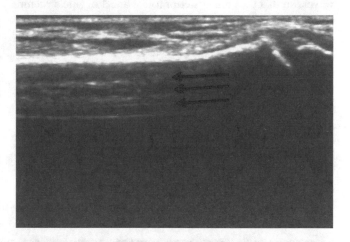

Fig. 2.5 Reverbation effect (repetition artifact) at the distal radius. (©Ackermann and Eckert 2015; Courtesy of off label media)

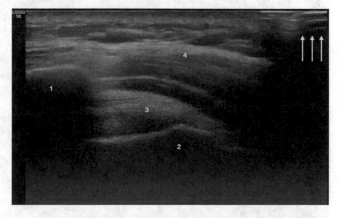

Fig. 2.6 Coupling artifact at the right edge of the image during lateral longitudinal section at the shoulder. 1 = Acromion, 2 = Humeral head, 3 = Supraspinatus tendon, 4 = M. deltoideus. (©Ackermann and Eckert 2015; Courtesy of off label media)

tion plane above the AC joint in slim patients with prominent bony changes at the top of the acromioclavicular joint and examining the foot in the longitudinal and transverse imaging of the Achilles tendon.

2.3.3 Arc Artefact

If a strongly echogenic structure (e.g. puncture needle) is sounded in an echo-free area (e.g. liquid), the so-called arc artefact is created.

2.4 Posterior Acoustic Enhancement

A posterior acoustic enhancement occurs when sound waves are moving through an anechogenic structure. By passing this anechogenic structure, there is more energy left in the sound waves, so that the area posterior to the anechogenic structure occurs with increased echogenic than the surrounding area.

For example in cysts, ganglia or fluid-filled cavities such as the gallbladder (Fig. 2.7).

2.5 Acoustic Shadowing

Acoustic shadowing refers to decreased sound strength behind a highly reflective object. When hitting such an objective, the sound waves are fully reflected and cannot penetrate the solid structure so that commonly a shadow occurs posterior to the object.

Bone surfaces, corresponding calcareous forms of the tendinosis calcarea (Fig. 2.8) or free joint bodies are classic examples of structures that cause acoustic shadowing.

2.6 Documentation

In addition to the obligatory details such as patient first and last name and date of birth, the examination date and time should also be documented for later reproducibility. While

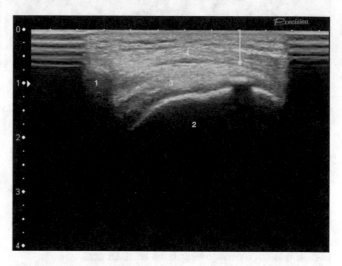

Fig. 2.8 Dorsal sound cancellation in case of tendinosis calcarea in the supraspinatus tendon in lateral longitudinal section. Secondary findings: Coupling artifacts on the left and right image margin in a very slim patient. 1 = Acromion, 2 = Humeral head, 3 = Supraspinatus tendon, 4 = M. deltoideus. (©Ackermann and Eckert 2015; Courtesy of off label media)

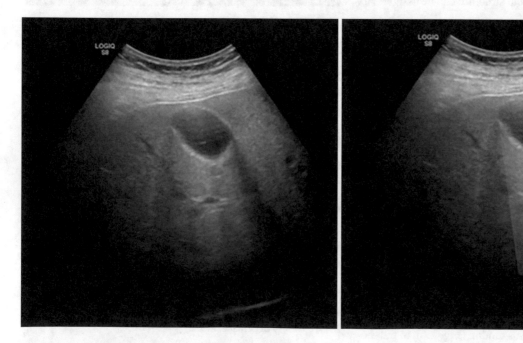

Fig. 2.7 Dorsal sound amplification behind the gall bladder. (©Ackermann and Eckert 2015; Courtesy of off label media)

the patient data must usually be entered manually or called up via a worklist, the date and time should generally be documented automatically and up to date with modern ultrasound equipment.

Furthermore, the ultrasound image must show the localization (which bone, which side) and the respective projection. In contrast to adult soft-tissue sonography, which requires findings to be made in at least two planes, the fracture sonography should be made from at least three projection planes, and if anatomically possible from four projections.

An electronic storage medium is recommended for the documentation; the thermal paper printouts used in the first-generation ultrasound devices are susceptible to mechanical damage, fade over time and are significantly more expensive overall. For those reasons, digital backup and archiving are recommended as the images can quickly and easily reproduce the condition at the time of examination in unaltered quality. Furthermore, it is advantageous in the clinical process for the post-treatment practitioner or examiner if the images are stored digitally in the central system and are easily accessible.

When adjusting the ultrasound image, care should be taken to ensure that the cortex is adjusted parallel to the upper edge of the monitor and across the entire width of the image. If there is an axial kinking in case of a fracture, the apex of the kink should be in the middle of the image. Near the joint, the corresponding epiphysis must also be shown. Otherwise, the same rules apply with regard to the orientation of ultrasound images as so far: the upper edge of the monitor is near the transducer, the lower edge of the monitor is far from the transducer, the left edge of the monitor is proximal and lateral (or radial and fibular) and the right edge of the monitor is distal and medial (or ulnar and tibial).

When documenting and archiving the findings and the images, there are a few things to consider. In contrast to conventional X-rays, in which the examined skeletal area can be clearly identified and the side is also marked accordingly, the ultrasound image does not allow the bony structure or the side to be identified. In order to avoid having to manually insert the corresponding parameters for each individual documented image, a structured, standardized and thus comprehensible examination procedure is recommended, which should be strictly adhered to for each examination. Only using this technique it is possible to draw conclusions about the position of the transducer head and thus the corresponding sectional plane on the basis of the available images. As an example, the examination procedure at the wrist (wrist-SAFE), in which the first picture is made dorsally over the distal radius, the second picture is 90° offset to the side of the radius, the next picture is again 90° offset from palmar over

the radius and so on. Based on the sequence of images, the exact section plane can be reproduced and evaluated afterwards (Fig. 2.9).

If an additional picture is made deviating from the defined standard examination, it must be marked accordingly.

2.7 Image Editing

At the beginning of diagnostics, the image conditions should be set and adjusted accordingly in order to get an optimized ultrasound image.

The frequency setting should be adapted to the soft tissue sheath around the bone, i.e. a higher frequency (i.e. high resolution at the surface, low penetration depth) should be selected if there is little soft tissue above the examined bone, while the frequency can be reduced (i.e. higher penetration depth, lower resolution) if the muscular sheath is thicker, such as on the thigh. Next, the focus position is adjusted to the height of the cortex to concentrate the optimal image sharpness to this area. Many modern ultrasound devices allow the number of focuses to be increased, but this slows down the repetition frequency and is usually not necessary in fracture sonography. Furthermore, the current devices allow scrolling back the last few seconds after 'freezing' the image (the length of this time varies depending on the manufacturer), usually with a trackball attached to the device, so the examiner can select the best image. This function is particularly useful in the sonography in children, as in the case of motion blur at the time of image freezing, the ultrasound image can be scrolled back step by step until a good image result can be achieved.

If the transducer is too small to fully document a pathological finding, there are two possibilities to combine individual images into a single image. Depending on the device a so-called sono-scan can be performed. In this case, after activating the function on the ultrasound device, the transducer is moved in a fluid motion over the region to be examined. The device automatically saves the ultrasound images at predefined time intervals and merges them into a complete single image when the function is terminated. A second option is to manually combine two ultrasound images. In this case, the screen is split at the touch of a button so that a complete transducer width is now displayed on each half of the monitor.

Even if diagnostically valuable and impressive images can be created in this way, it should always be kept in mind that ultrasound diagnostics is a two-dimensional imaging technique, even if the images can sometimes give a three-dimensional impression due to the above-mentioned modern partly automatic processing possibilities.

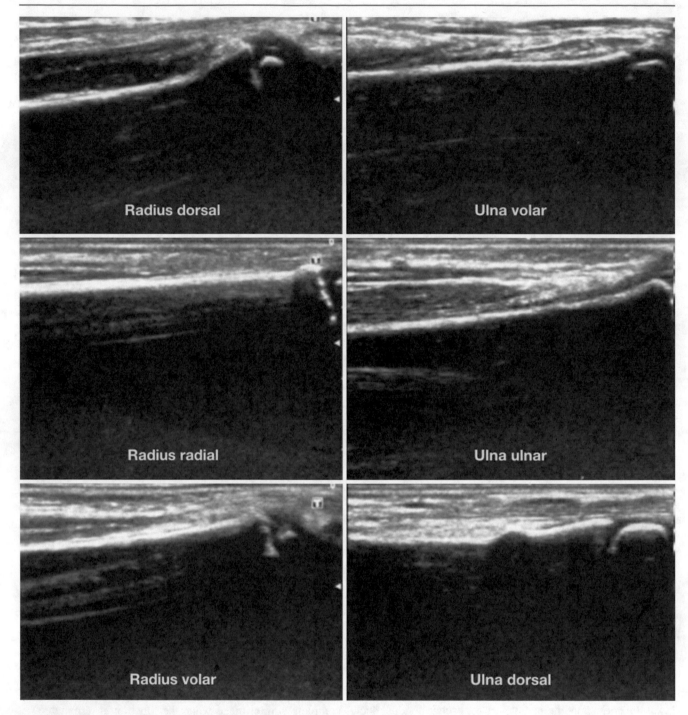

Fig. 2.9 Wrist SAFE documentation. (©Ackermann and Eckert 2015; Courtesy of off label media)

2.8 Pseudo-fractures in the Ultrasound Image

Ole Ackermann

There are various artefacts and findings in sonographic diagnostics that can be incorrectly interpreted as fractures:

2.8.1 Epiphyseal Hook

There is often a small hook-shaped structure on the shaft-side epiphyseal plate, which can be mistaken for a fracture, but is physiological. With increasing experience in fracture sonography, especially by examining healthy patients, the examiner learns to safely differentiate the epiphyseal hook from fractures (Figs. 2.10, 2.11, 2.12, and 2.13).

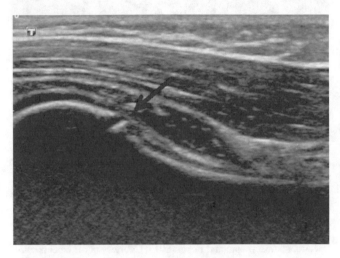

Fig 2.10 Humerus left, a.p.-Projection; arrow: epiphyseal hook. (©Ackermann and Eckert 2015; Courtesy of off label media)

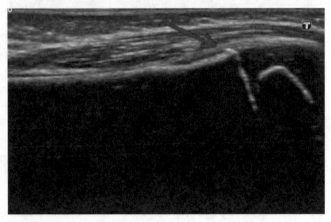

Fig. 2.12 Distal radius, dorsal projection: torus fracture; arrow: Epiphysel hook. (©Ackermann and Eckert 2015; Courtesy of off label media)

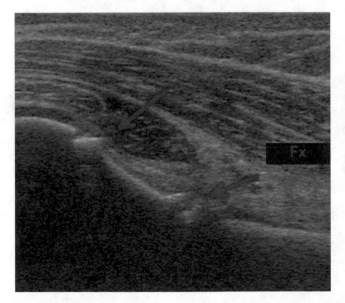

Fig. 2.11 Proximal humerus, a.-p. Projection; left arrow: epiphyseal hook; right arrow: fracture. (©Ackermann and Eckert 2015; Courtesy of off label media)

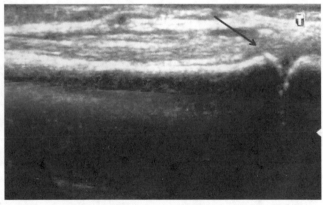

Fig. 2.13 Distal radius, dorsal projection; arrow: Epiphyseal hook. (©Ackermann and Eckert 2015; Courtesy of off label media)

2.8.2 Pseudo Fracture/Deletion

If the ultrasonic waves run parallel to the surface of the bone, no echo is reflected and in this area there is sound cancellation, which can be mistaken for a fracture. This effect often arises at the point of transition from the convex to the concave bend on the fossa olecrani or at the rounding of epiphyseal cores. These artefacts can be identified by changing the display level (Figs. 2.14 and 2.15).

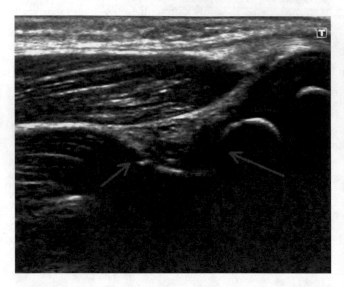

Fig. 2.14 Fossa olecrani, dorsal longitudinal view; arrows: deletion, no fractures. (©Ackermann and Eckert 2015; Courtesy of off label media)

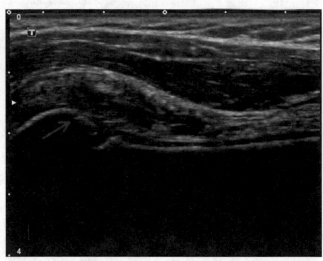

Fig. 2.15 Proximal humerus, ventral projection; arrow: deletion, no fracture. (©Ackermann and Eckert 2015; Courtesy of off label media)

Part II
Special Indications

Skullcap

3

Axel Feldkamp

3.1 Synopsis

1.1 **Rationale of application:** X-ray-free diagnosis of dome fractures.
1.2 **Level of evidence:** Ia.
1.3 **Indication:** X-ray-free diagnosis if skullcap fracture is suspected, especially if there is a distinctly external marker (hematoma).
1.4 **Contraindications:**
   - open fractures.
   - neurological abnormalities.
   - suspected fracture of the viscerocranium.
   - suspected fracture of the skull base.
1.5 **Age of the patient:** 0–18 years.
1.6 **Examination:** Representation in the plane across the fracture. Examine the fracture along this plane to determine the extent. The representation in the plane of the fracture expansion is not successful.
1.7 **Indications for additional imaging:**
   - uncertainty in the assessment.
   - neurological abnormalities.
   - suspected intracranial injuries.
   - unconsciousness.
1.8 **Pitfalls:**
   - open skull sutures.
   - external hematomas and mirror image (artifact).
   - connatal impression of the skullcap.
   - system disorders.
1.9 **Red flags:**
   - see above.

A. Feldkamp (✉)
Sana Kliniken AG, Klinikum Duisburg, Duisburg, Germany
e-mail: axel.feldkamp@sana.de

3.2 Introduction

Traumatic brain injury (TBI) is a common childhood injury. About 28% of all TBI affects patients under the age of 16. In Germany, this age group assumes 581 patients per 100.000 inhabitants. Only less than 10% can be classified as moderate or severe TBI. Exact numbers of cases for the skull fracture are not known.

Sonography is a very good method for imaging such a skull fracture. The analysis of several studies showed a sensitivity of 88% and a specificity of 97% for sonography. However, it should be noted that these very good results relate to fractures of the skull cap. Midface fractures and, of course, skull base fractures can be diagnosed significantly poorly or not by sonography [2, 3, 4, 5].

The calotte fracture is only one possible injury in a TBI. Bleeding and injuries of the brain and intracerebral vessels are more serious. Here, especially with closed fontanel sonography is not a method with sufficient certainty (compare third indications and fourth contraindications).

3.3 Indication

The indication for fracture sonography is the suspicion or the exclusion of a skull fracture. In principle, any child with a traumatic brain injury can be sonographed, but this does not seem to make sense. It makes no sense to search the entire calotte for a fracture. This would be relatively time-consuming and would not make sense if there were no indications of a fracture. However, there are anamnestic and clinical signs that make fracture more likely in traumatic brain injury. A circumscribed region of the head can then be examined in a targeted manner.

Possiblve indications include:

- a circumscribed soft tissue swelling
- a hematoma (bump mark)

- a circumscribed pressure pain
- safe localization of the effects of violence in the event of adequate trauma

The sonography is then carried out specifically at these points. Fractures beyond such regions are very rare.

However, the contraindications and indications for CT or MRI diagnostics (see below) must be taken into account. Particularly in the case of neurological abnormalities, the question of intracerebral injuries is in the foreground, so that the pure fracture detection is not indicative.

3.4 Contraindications and Indications to Other Imaging Procedures

There is a contraindication for using sonography in case of open injuries because of causing additional pain and possible infection by ultrasound gel.

Cranial CT is still considered the gold standard in patients with skull injuries. The focus is not on the question of the fracture but rather the question of intracranial injuries. Due to the radiation exposure to the child, the indication must be set much more strictly than in adult medicine. In this regard, MRI would be preferable; it also has a higher sensitivity for circumscribed tissue lesions. Due to the high expenditure on equipment, the time required and the frequent need for sedation or anesthesia in smaller children, it is currently often not an option as a primary imaging method. It should also be borne in mind here that proper neurological monitoring after anesthesia is not possible.

Sonography can be used to address intracranial injury. This is done transfontanellar (Figs. 3.1 and 3.2), older children must be examined transcranial. However, an inconspicuous examination does not rule out space-consuming hemorrhage near the dome. Bleeding or injuries in the posterior cranial fossa are not adequately recorded.

The mandatory indications for performing cranial CT are:

- coma
- persistent loss of consciousness
- focal neurological disorders (paresis, cranial nerve failure, cerebral attack)
- suspected impression fracture, skull base fracture, and open injuries

Optional indications are:

- serious accident mechanism (e.g., car accident, fall height > 1.5 m, unclear anamnesis)
- severe or persistent headache
- vomiting with a close temporal relationship to the effects of violence and in the event of repeated occurrence
- intoxication with alcohol or drugs
- if there is evidence of a clotting disorder [1]

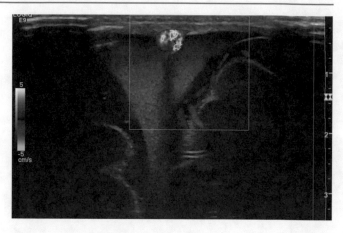

Fig. 3.1 Coronal section through the fontanel. More echogenic blood on both sides in the subdural space. The subarachnoid space is less echogenic; it can be identified in the color Doppler examination using the pervasive vessels (bridge veins)

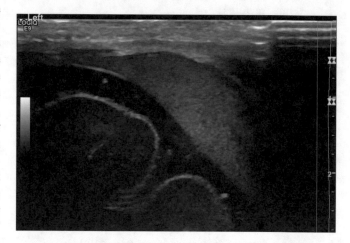

Fig. 3.2 Sagittal section through the fontanel. Lower echogenic subarachnoid space above the gyri, pulling into the sulci. Above that is the more echogenic subdural space

If an impression fracture is diagnosed sonographically, additional imaging (CT or MRI) should follow. This is also necessary for the indication of an operation.

3.5 Investigation

After taking the medical history and the clinical examination, including a neurological assessment, the sonographic examination follows. This includes the examination of the skullcap; in case of open fontanel, the intracranial finding should always be ascertained.

3.5.1 Technical Requirements

Due to the curved shape of the head, a lot of gel is usually necessary to achieve a good coupling of the linear transducer. Depending on hair growth, a lot of gel is also necessary to avoid air artifacts (sound cancellation). This is sometimes a real challenge with very curly hair.

3.5.2 Positioning

Special storage is not necessary. The child should be supine on the examination table. The head only needs to be examined in the lateral or prone position in occipital fractures. The head does not have to be fixed, as a rule the examiner can compensate for minor head movements with the transducer. It must be ensured that pressure with the transducer should be avoided, especially the bouncing mark can be painful. Another reason not to save with gel.

3.5.3 Section Plane

There is no defined section plane. Furthermore, it is not possible to systematically search the entire calotte for a fracture. Therefore, the ultrasound examination should be carried out in the region of the clinically conspicuous region. The clinically noticeable region of the head is:

– soft tissue swelling
– hematoma
– point of violence (if known)
– point of maximum pressure pain

The transducer is placed in this area with a lot of gel without pressure.

A fracture can only be displayed if the plane of the ultrasound section crosses the plane of the fracture. This means that a representation parallel to the fracture line is not possible. For this reason, the region examined must be represented in at least two mutually perpendicular planes. To do this, the entire region must be surveyed in these levels by moving the transducer.

The few false-negative results in the studies were almost all due to fractures that were not in the region of the study.

Fractures are to be differentiated from open skull sutures; a morphological differentiation is not possible (see Sect. 3.6).

3.5.4 Setting

If the fracture is found using the above procedure, the course of the fracture gap must be shown by moving the transducer. Once the course has been clarified, the transducer must be turned so that the formwork level is set at 90° to the fracture line. The fracture can only be assessed precisely at this level (width of the fracture gap, position of the fragments relative to one another).

The fracture gap must then be screened completely. To do this, move the transducer in both directions along the fracture gap. Only in this way it is possible to determine the course and length of the fracture gap.

A statement about the width of the fracture gap and the existence of a step formation is only permitted if the fracture has been examined over the entire length of the fracture line. Clips are very helpful for documentation [4].

3.5.5 Assessment and Diagnosis

Only the outer boundary of the calotte (external tabula) can be shown in ultrasound, since there are total reflection and absorption of the sound waves at the interface of the bone. In the case of a fracture, this interface is interrupted and the fracture gap is shown as a low echoic to anechoic interruption (Fig. 3.3).

This type of skull fracture shows a very good correlation with corresponding CT examinations (Figs. 3.4 and 3.5).

The width of the fracture gap can be determined, but is of minor importance. If the fracture gap is very wide, it is often possible to identify the underlying brain structures. With a very wide fracture gap, a prolapse of brain tissue can occur in rare cases. Here, the fracture gap is filled with inhomogeneous tissue, which can be tracked continuously extra- and intracranially (Fig. 3.6).

Dome fractures are complicated by displacement of the fragments. This creates a step. The fragments are shifted against each other or can overlap. The difference in height of the two fragments can be determined sonographically (Figs. 3.7 and 3.8). An intracranial injury can be expected to a greater extent in both types of dome fracture, so that further imaging should generally follow.

The impression fracture can be recognized as another form. Here, fragments of the fracture are shifted inwards, i.e., toward the brain. Such a fracture must always result in further imaging, since there is a high degree of intracranial bleeding.

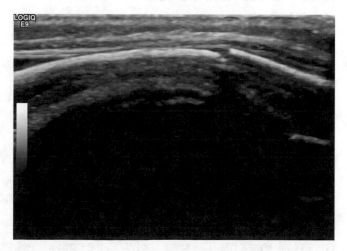

Fig. 3.3 Representation of the low echoic interruption of the otherwise rich echoic skull cap. The periosteum appears intact

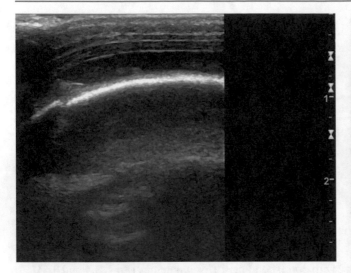

Fig. 3.4 Narrow fracture gap with minimal displacement of the fragments

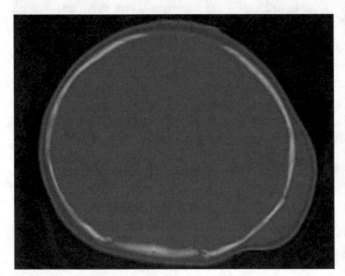

Fig. 3.5 Corresponding CT examination

3.5.6 Therapy and Controls

Therapy depends more on the intracranial finding. A non-displaced fracture in a neurologically unremarkable child does not require specific therapy and control. Further imaging should be performed for all fractures with fragment displacement. The indication for therapy then results from the relevant findings.

3.6 Pitfalls and Red Flags

3.6.1 Open Skull Sutures

In newborns, the fontanelles are still open; the ossification takes place over time. The same applies to the skull sutures. There are no standard values for the width of the fontanelles and skull sutures, there is a large variance here.

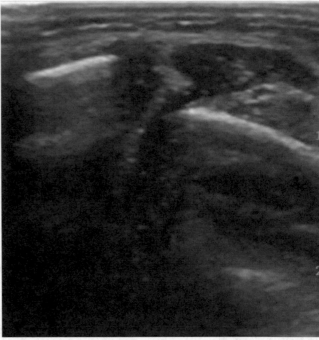

Fig. 3.6 Wide dome fracture with evidence of prolapsed brain tissue (Fig. by J. Jüngert, Erlangen)

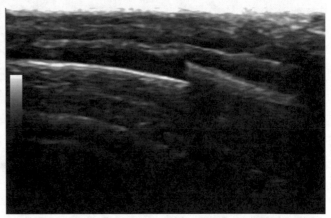

Fig. 3.7 Skull fracture. The fragments show a step formation and are shifted one above the other (Fig. by G. Schweintzger, Leoben Austria)

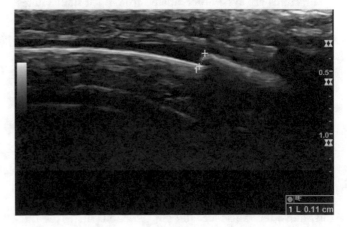

Fig. 3.8 Same fracture with determination of the height difference of the fragments (Fig. by G. Schweintzger, Leoben Austria)

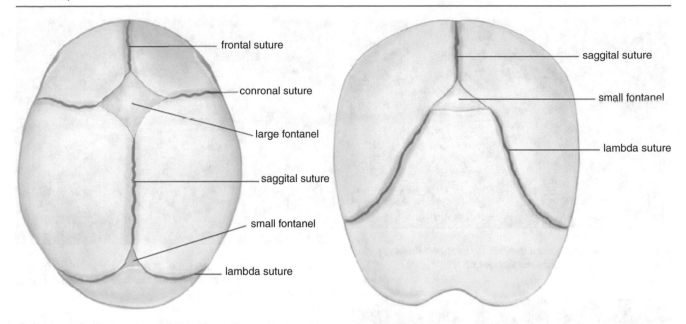

Figs. 3.9 and 3.10 Sketch of the skull sutures from above sketch of the skull sutures from behind

The bony closure also varies, mostly the fontanelles and sutures can no longer be displayed from the age of 1. In some cases, however, the presentation succeeds beyond the second year of life. The frontal seam can be closed much earlier.

Open skull sutures cannot be distinguished sonographically from fractures. Knowledge of the course of the skull sutures is therefore necessary (Figs. 3.9 and 3.10).

The coronary suture (coronary suture, sutura coronalis) lies between the os frontale and os parietale on both sides, the sagittal suture (sutura sagittalis) lies between the two ossa parietalis and the lambda suture (sutura lambdoidea) lies between the os occipitale and the os parietale also on both sides.

Since open skull sutures cannot be reliably distinguished from fractures in terms of their image morphology, other criteria must be used. Sagittal, frontal, and coronary suture can be traced to the edge of the large fontanelle, the lambda suture to the small fontanelle (Fig. 3.11). Furthermore, when in doubt, the side comparison for the paired coronary and lambda sutures is helpful.

3.6.2 External Hematomas and Mirror Artifacts

Large-scale extracranial hematomas often occur after childbirth. Fractures are rare. Since such hematomas often only appear days to weeks after birth, the question of a fracture often arises.

The hematomas can be clearly differentiated with regard to their location using sonography. First, the hematomas appear differently echogenic depending on the extent. As they progress, they become increasingly low-echo or anechoic.

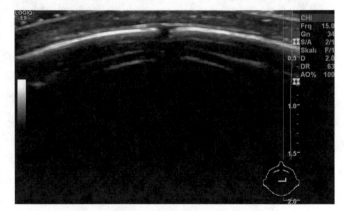

Fig. 3.11 Representation of the open coronary suture

The caput succedaneum is located between the scalp and the galea aponeurotica. Therefore, they can cross the skull sutures. The same applies to the subgaleal hematoma, which is located between the aponeurotica and the periosteum.

In this respect, the cephalic hematoma lies between the periosteum and the bone, such a hematoma does not exceed the sutures of the skull (Fig. 3.12).

An echo-free structure, which is often confused with an epidural hematoma (Fig. 3.13), often also appears below these echo-free fluid collections below the calotte boundary layer. It is a mirror artifact, so a structure below the calotte is only "mirrored."

3.6.3 Connatal Cranial Impression

Newborns have a thin skullcap and open skull sutures. This provides the prerequisite for passage through the maternal pel-

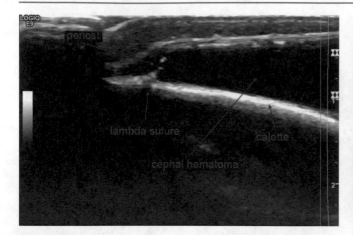

Fig. 3.12 Cephalic hematoma showing the location below the periosteum. It does not exceed the open skull suture

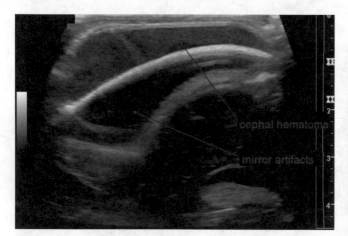

Fig. 3.13 Mirror artifact in case of a cephal hematoma

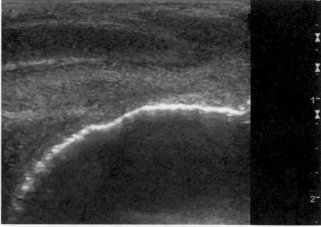

Fig. 3.14 Illustration of indentation of the calotte without a fracture gap. Significant swelling above the calotte. It is a connective cranial impression after forceps delivery

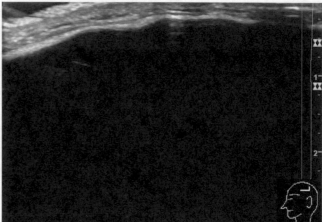

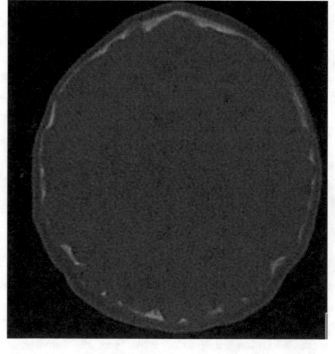

Figs. 3.15 and 3.16 Irregular skullcap in Crouzon's disease corresponding CT image

vis. Nevertheless, skull impressions occur in 1–2.5 per 10,000 births. Such impressions often arise without a fracture, they are also known as ping-pong deformities. These are similar to greenstick-like fractures of the extremities with preserved periosteum. Seventy percent arise frontally, 30% parietally.

The impression (indentation) can be displayed sonographically, a fracture line is missing (Fig. 3.14).

3.6.4 Systemic Diseases

There are a number of diseases with defects or thinning of the calotte. These include histiocytosis X and neurofibromatosis, mostly with multiple defects. In Crouzon's disease, premature sutures lead to pressure marks (thinning) of the calotte with clear irregularities in the bone surface (Figs. 3.15 and 3.16) in the sonographic image. Confusion with fractures and impressions is rare, however, since there is generally no history of trauma, a corresponding hematoma is missing, and the children have further stigmas.

References

AWMF Leitlinie: Das Schädel-Hirn-Trauma im Kindesalter

1. www.awmf.org/uploads/tx_szleitlinien/024-018l_S2k_Schaedel-Hirn-Trauma_im_Kindesalter-2011-abgelaufen.pdf.awmf.sht.kindesalter.

Accurary of Point-of-Care Ultrasound for Diagnosis of Skull Fractures in Children

2. Rabiner JE, Friedman LM, Khine H, Avner JR, Tsung JW. Pediatrics. 2013;131(6):1757–64.

Accuracy of Clinician-Performed Point-of-Care Ultrasound for the Diagnosis of Fractures in Children and Young Adults

3. Weinberg ER, Tunik MG, Tsung JW. Injury. 2010;41(8):862–8.

Ability of Emergency Ultrasonography to Detect Pediatric Skull Fractures in Children: A Prospective, Observational Study

4. Parri N, Crosby BJ, Glass C, et al. J Emerg Med. 2013;44(1):135–41.

Ultrasound Evaluation of Skull Fractures in Children: A Feasibility Study

5. Riera A, Chen L. Pediatr Emerg Care. 2012;28(5):420–5.

Fractures of the Clavicle

4

Hartmut Gaulrapp

4.1 Synopsis

1.1 Rationale of application: X-ray-free diagnosis of clavicle fractures in newborns and children.
1.2 Evidence level: IIa.
1.3 Indication: Imaging diagnostics for suspected clavicular fractures in newborns and children.
1.4 Contraindications: open fractures, complex thoracic traumas.
1.5 Age of the patient: 0–15 years.
1.6 Examination: Sections along the clavicle, starting anterior, then moving the transducer cranially for the second level.
1.7 Indications for additional X-ray diagnostics:
   – Significant step formation or side shift.
   – Vascular or nerval symptoms.
   – uncertainty in the assessment.
   – recurrent fractures.
1.8 Pitfalls:
   – complex traumas.
   – battered child syndrome.
   – systemic diseases (e.g., osteogenesis imperfecta).
1.9 Red flags:
   – severe pain/immobility without proof of fracture.
   – fracture without adequate trauma.
   – pre-traumatic complaints at this location.
   – recurrent fractures.
   – increasing complaints under therapy.
   – family history of relevant systemic diseases.

4.2 Introduction

Clavicle fractures are the most common form of fracture at the shoulder girdle in childhood. In newborns they can be the result of the birth process. In walking children, they occur as a result of falls. The diagnosis can be made sonographically in the children's emergency room after minimal instruction.

4.3 Indication

Swelling in the area of the clavicle after birth, especially after pulling the arm or compressing the shoulder girdle, can immediately be clarified by the use of ultrasonography. Older children usually present themselves in the ambulance after a fall on the hand or against a wall with pain in the anterior shoulder area.

4.4 Indications for X-ray Diagnostics

Open injuries, other co-injured structures on the thorax, especially in suspected cases of child abuse.

4.5 Investigation

4.5.1 Patient's Positioning

Newborns are hold by the child's nurse keeping their head to the opposite side. Older children can sit on a relative's lap or by their own. Small children, in particular, sometimes resist the ultrasound examination for fear. The examination itself is painless.

H. Gaulrapp (✉)
Facharztpraxis für Orthopädie, Kinder-Orthopädie und Sportmedizin, Munich, Germany

© Springer Nature Switzerland AG 2021
O. Ackermann (ed.), *Fracture Sonography*, https://doi.org/10.1007/978-3-030-63839-9_4

4.5.2 Section Levels

The clavicle is examined from anterior to cranial in longitudinally directed sections to the bone, including the adjacent sternal as well as the acromial joint.

4.5.3 Setting

Due to their curved shape and the low subcutaneous tissue coverage, both the scanning process with the transducer and the image acquisition in the unfavorable near focus area are sometimes difficult. Increased contact pressure can be painful and make the examination even more difficult.

4.5.4 Assessment

Compared to an X-ray ultrasonography can accurately detect clavicular fractures in newborns, so that the connection between clinical and sonographic diagnostics is sufficient for diagnosis and documentation. It is also the first imaging method in older children after trauma, but also in case of unclear pain localization, then followed by a targeted X-ray image of the sonographically predefined region.

If the clavicle is bruised, an echo-poor periosteal hematoma can be found sonographically as a sign of the bleeding (Fig. 4.1). A crack is characterized by an interruption in the echogenic bone line (Fig. 4.2a and b). Step formation can be assessed both sonographically and in the X-ray image (Fig. 4.3a and b).

4.5.5 Diagnosis

The goal of sonographic examination is to visualize periosteal hemorrhage or an interruption of the echogenic bone contour. This justifies the diagnosis of a collarbone fracture. Kink formation can be detected easily, step formation or shifts by shaft width are more difficult to record and document in a single image.

4.5.6 Therapy and Controls

Depending on the age of the injured child, bone-healing signs can be recognized sonographically 1 week before the appearance on the X-ray (Fig. 4.4a and b). After 7 days, a newborn fracture shows a periosteal reaction, after 10 days, the callus formation

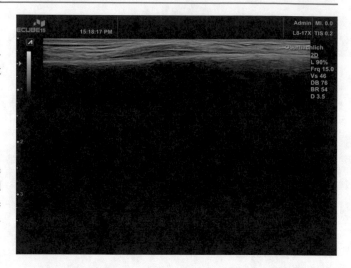

Fig. 4.1 Six-year-old patient after bruise: periosteal hematoma

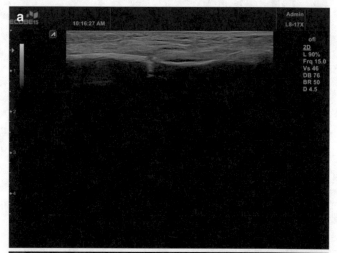

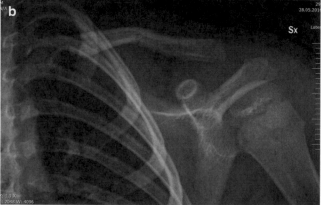

Fig. 4.2 (**a**) Five-year-old patient with fissure: break in the bone line and slight kink in the sonogram. (**b**) X-ray image of (**a**) with slight kinking as in the sonogram

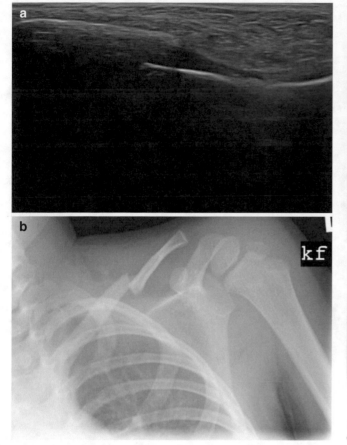

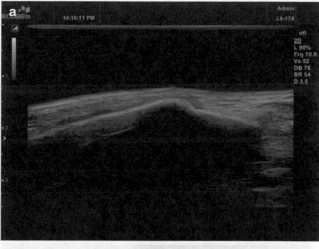

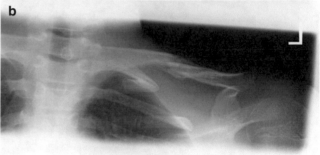

Fig. 4.4 (**a**) 11-year-old patient 4 weeks after fracture with a broad, echogenic bone line. (**b**) X-ray image for (**a**)

Fig. 4.3 (**a**) Patient with typical central fracture and step formation. (**b**) X-ray image of (**a**) also shows the step formation

begins, which can have several layers through the course of time and may be more pronounced in younger children. After 20 days, bridging shows up and after 35 days extensive remodeling. Since sonography precedes the X-ray image and complete remodeling plays no role for load-bearing, X-ray can be replaced by sonography in the follow-up of pediatric fractures.

Knowledge of the healing signs of the bone is particularly important when child abuse is suspected in order to determine the time period of the past injury.

4.6   Pitfalls and Red Flags

In the case of complex thoracic trauma, other structures have priority. Clavicular fractures can be identified by a whole-body CT performed in the shock room. Etiologically incomprehensible injuries must always be thought of as a hint to a battered child syndrome. Repeated osseous injuries could indicate systemic diseases, e.g., osteogenesis imperfecta.

In the case of severe pain without a history of fractures, an X-ray must be taken instead of an ultrasound, possibly also an MRI.

Further Reading

1. Assafiri I, Sraj S. Adolescent displaced midshaft clavicle fracture. J Hand Surg Am. 2015;40:145–7. https://doi.org/10.1016/j.jhsa.2014.09.023. Epub 2014 Oct 23.
2. Bartoli E, Saporetti N, Marchetti S. Ruolo dell' ecografia nella diagnosi della fratture clavicolari del neonato. Radiol Med. 1989;77:466–9.
3. Blab E, Geissler W, Rokitansky A. Sonographic management of infantile clavicular fractures. Pediatr Surg Int. 1999;15:251–4.
4. Chien M, Bulloch B, Garcia-Filion P, Youssfi M, Shrader MW, Segal LS. Bedside ultrasound in the diagnosis of pediatric clavicle fractures. Pediatr Emerg Care. 2011;27:1038–41.
5. Cross KP, Warkentine FH, Kim IK, Gracely E, Paul RI. Bedside ultrasound diagnosis of clavicle fractures in the pediatric emergency department. Acad Emerg Med. 2010;17:687–93.
6. Fadell M, Miller A, Trefan L, Weinman J, Stewart J, Hayes K, Maguire S. Radiological features of healing in newborn clavicular fractures. Eur Radiol. 2017;27:2180–7.
7. Katz R, Landman J, Dulitzky F, Bar-Ziv J. Fracture of the clavicle in the newborn. An ultrasound diagnosis. J Ultrasound Med. 1988;7:21–3.
8. Kayser R, Mahlfeld K, Heyde C, Grasshoff H. Ultrasonographic imaging of fractures of the clavicle in newborn infants. J Bone Joint Surg Br. 2003;85:115–6.
9. Moritz JD, Berthold LD, Soenksen SF, Alzen GF. Ultrasound in diagnosis of fractures in children: unnecessary harassment or useful addition to X-ray? Ultraschall Med. 2008;29:267–74.

Acromioclavicular Joint Instability

5

Hans-Jürgen Kock

5.1 Synopsis

1.1 **Rationale of application**: X-ray-free evaluation of injuries to the acromioclavicular (AC) joint with instability according to both the Tossy and the Rockwood classification.

1.2 **Level of evidence**: II.

1.3 **Indication**: Suspected stable and unstable shoulder joint injuries.

1.4 **Contraindications**: Accompanying open fractures, suspected vascular or nerve damage, clearly visible dislocation with a surgical indication.

1.5 **Age of the patient**: 16–75 years.

1.6 **Examination**: First, orienting ultrasound examination on the uninjured side in the frontal plane, sagittal plane, and horizontal plane without weight bearing and then possibly with weight bearing of up to 10 kg. Then the identical examination on the injured side in the same order. Image documentation always in comparison to the contralateral uninjured side in all planes.

1.7 **Indications for additional radiographic evaluation**: Suspected lateral clavicular fractures or other concomitant bony injuries that cannot be correctly assessed or excluded by ultrasound.

1.8 **Pitfalls**:
- lateral clavicular fractures
- humeral head fractures and humeral head dislocations
- rib fractures
- non-dislocated and dislocated epiphyseal injuries.

1.9 **Red flags**: Severe pain and/or immobility without evidence of fracture without demonstration of AC joint instability.

H.-J. Kock (✉)
MEDIAN Hohenfeld Klinik, Bad Camberg, Germany
e-mail: kock.da@t-online.de,
hans-juergen.kock@median-kliniken.de

5.2 Introduction

Injuries to the acromioclavicular (AC) joint are among the most common injuries in the area of the shoulder girdle. The injuries are traditionally classified worldwide according to radiographic criteria in the classifications of Tossy and more recently of Rockwood. In Europe, Tossy III injuries are mostly treated with surgery, whereas until recently these injuries were mostly not operated on in the United States.

After the historical beginnings in the German-speaking world in the late 1980s, in the 1990s, the use of ultrasound for the evaluation of vertical instability in acromioclavicular joint injuries spread worldwide. For around 20 years, ultrasound examination of the acromioclavicular joint has been used by various examiners initially for the parallel evaluation of soft tissue damage in Tossy injuries of type I–III [1–5]. These first publications demonstrated early on that acromioclavicular joint ultrasonography which, for scientific reasons, was initially generally carried out with radiographic controls for validation, was a very reliable and easily learned examination technique.

Even if the beginnings of AC joint ultrasound go back a long way, through the internationalization of examination techniques, along with the clinical expansion from the Tossy classification to the Rockwood classification, the clinical relevance of ultrasonographic and radiographic examinations became increasingly complex.

In a recent meta-analysis of the scientific studies published to date on this clinically relevant topic (surgical indication for Tossy III injury versus conservative therapy for Tossy II instability), Pogorzelski et al. 2017 [6] again show that the distinction between type III and type V injuries according to the Rockwood classification is still controversial. In addition, the Rockwood Type VI injury is such a rare entity that its inclusion in a classification has recently been questioned by some experts [7].

Until the final clarification of this problem by means of appropriate prospective randomized studies, the examination of acromioclavicular joint instability should be carried

© Springer Nature Switzerland AG 2021
O. Ackermann (ed.), *Fracture Sonography*, https://doi.org/10.1007/978-3-030-63839-9_5

out both vertically and horizontally using reliable and reproducible methods. In this context, the value of the universally available X-ray examinations which can be carried out in a standardized manner must be emphasized once again.

Appropriate imaging for objective documentation of AC joint instabilities should also always be performed before unclear surgical indications.

As things currently stand, on the basis of evaluation of the publications available in the literature [6–12], the following procedure can be recommended:

5.2.1 Assessment of Vertical Instability

In contrast to radiographic and above all ultrasound evaluation of horizontal stability, the value of which has not yet been conclusively demonstrated, numerous studies since the 1980s have shown ultrasound examination of vertical stability to be very reliable and quite easily performed.

In a recent review [6], 13 papers were examined for their reliability and consistently showed good or very good results. Ultrasound can differentiate reliably between sprain and rupture of the AC and CC (coracoclavicular) ligaments. The contralateral comparison enables classification using an AC joint index analogous to the Tossy classification [3]. Both the inter- and intra-observer reliability for this standardized radiographic evaluation of the vertical instability of the clavicle in the AC joint showed a high degree of reproducibility with mostly good to very good results [6].

However, the authors of the publications available to date point out that clavicular films in two planes are still required to ensure definite radiographic exclusion of fractures.

5.2.2 Assessment of Horizontal Instability

In a recent literature search of 1359 publications, 17 studies were selected that met the inclusion criteria for a literature search using the Cochrane methodology [6]. Of these 17 selected studies, 12 dealt with examination of vertical instability (see above) using X-ray imaging. It should be emphasized that in all these studies radiographic examination for exclusion of fractures was considered necessary.

This is probably the reason why the algorithms available to date indicate the superiority of X-ray evaluation over acromioclavicular joint ultrasonography for the evaluation of horizontal instability, especially since the use of ultrasound for evaluation of horizontal instability has not yet been described in the literature.

In contrast to the sonographic evaluation of vertical AC joint instability [3, 6], which has been described for a long time, the visualization of horizontal instability appears to be technically and anatomically far more demanding and can therefore not currently be recommended.

5.2.3 Diagnostic Value of Weight-Bearing Examinations

The value of weight-bearing panorama studies with 10 kg weights in contralateral comparison has been debated worldwide for many decades [overview see [6]]. Toward the end of the 1980s, already, some authors were able to show that the comparison of panorama X-rays with and without weight bearing had no diagnostic value. Therefore, these authors recommended that these X-rays no longer be requested for patients due to the associated painfulness.

However, newer studies have only recently shown that the value of panorama views with 10-kg weights did lead to increased sensitivity with regard to the differentiation between Tossy II and Tossy III or between Rockwood III and IV instabilities.

Since only a few studies with good scientific reliability have been carried out on this topic, a final scientific assessment of the value of weight-bearing panorama X-rays is not yet possible.

5.3 Indication and Patient Age

Ultrasound examination of shoulder joint instability is indicated in patients with an appropriate accident history and typical clinical findings (tenderness over the AC joint and possibly "piano key phenomenon"), from adolescents to active seniors (approx. 16–75 years). The patients usually present with pain in the affected AC joint after direct trauma, e.g., after falling on the shoulder while riding a bicycle or during contact sports such as ice hockey, American football, or judo.

Despite the relative rarity of AC joint instabilities, which account for only 4% of injuries to the upper shoulder girdle, this injury requires a subtle examination technique with fracture exclusion through X-ray examinations of the clavicle in two planes and subsequent evaluation of instability with weight-bearing panorama images. Even if their value is ultimately still scientifically controversial, an initially diagnosed Tossy II injury can turn out to be a Tossy III lesion due to the tensile load.

The same applies to the ultrasound detection of AC joint instabilities, which can be objectified by comparison to the contralateral uninjured side using a so-called AC joint index [3].

5.4 Contraindications and Indications for X-ray Evaluation

All scientific studies on this topic indicate the importance of radiographic exclusion of clavicular fractures.

In addition, however, all authors point out the outstanding value of ultrasound examination for the evaluation of soft tissue damage and other accompanying injuries. In unclear situations, reliable diagnosis and classification of the degree of instability according to the Tossy classification can often be carried out by means of stress imaging with traction and countertraction compared to the contralateral uninjured side.

In all cases with suspected concomitant injury to the vessels and nerves, further diagnostic assessment is necessary, e.g., by requesting a CT scan or a magnetic resonance scan, if necessary also with contrast agent.

From our own clinical practice, it must be emphasized that inexperienced examiners are advised to perform an X-ray examination of the acromioclavicular joint instability before any operative therapy in order to be able to check the indication objectively and reproducibly at any time and in the long term.

5.5 Examination Procedure

It has proved useful to begin by examining the uninjured contralateral side in the seated patient first in the vertical plane and then in the sagittal plane using a linear transducer (5–10 MHz).

An ultrasound standoff with gel is usually not necessary. With the patient's arm hanging down, the opposite uninjured side is first examined in all three planes. Then the injured side is examined and the findings are documented. Finally, an extended instability assessment for Tossy/Rockwood classification is carried out on both arms with the patient holding 10-kg weights.

After a short learning phase, the examiner is able quickly and reliably to classify the instability compared to the uninjured contralateral side.

The examination is painless and can be carried out quickly. For the practiced examiner, the ultrasound examination of both sides takes about 5 min. The ultrasound evaluation of AC joint instability is thus an easy-to-learn entry-level examination in shoulder girdle ultrasonography.

5.5.1 Assessment

In addition to the width of the AC joint space, the extent of a hematoma can regularly be described. Occasionally, longer ligament ends or an intraarticular disc can be detected by ultrasound.

Determination of the CC distance is often possible in slim patients; determination of the AC distance is almost always possible even in obese patients.

For the ultrasound measurement of the AC distance as a direct measure of AC instability, the widest measurable distance between the acromial and the clavicular cortical margins of the bony structures of the joint is measured (see Fig. 5.1).

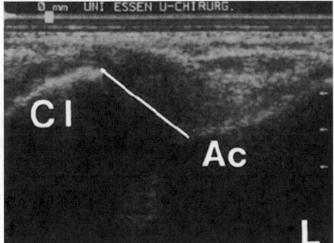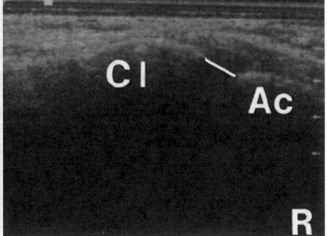

Fig. 5.1 Acromioclavicular joint sonography in a patient with a left Tossy III injury (7.5 MHz linear transducer). The sonographic measured AC joint width is 19 mm on the left (L = injured side) and 4 mm on the right (R = uninjured side). This results in the so-called AC joint index with 0.21 (=width of the uninjured side/width of the injured side). With a sonographically proven AC joint index of <0.3, a Tossy III injury can be assumed. *Cl* clavicle, *Ac* acromion. (From Kock et al. 1996)

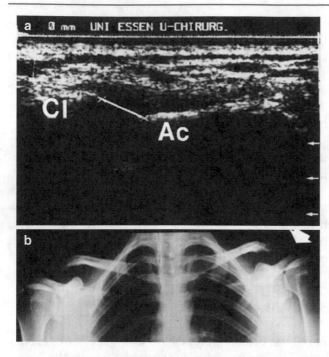

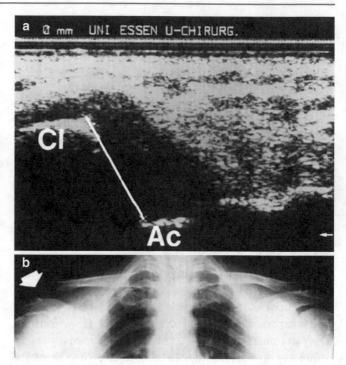

Fig. 5.2 (a) Shoulder corner joint sonography in a patient with a Tossy I injury on the left (7.5 MHz linear transducer). The sonographically measured AC joint width is left (=injured side) 5.1 mm and on the right (=unbroken side) 5.3 mm. This results in the so-called AC joint index with 0.96 (=width of the uninjured side/width the injured side). (b) Conventional X-ray panoramic image of the same patient. *Cl* clavicle, *Ac* acromion. (From Kock et al. 1996)

Fig. 5.4 (a) Acromioclavicular joint sonography in a patient with a Tossy III injury on the left (7.5 MHz linear transducer). The sonographically measured AC joint width is left (=injured side) 24 mm and on the right (=non-injured side) 3 mm. Calculated from this the so-called AC joint index is 0.13 (=width of the uninjured side/width of the injured side). (b) Conventional panoramic image of the same patient. *Cl* clavicle, *Ac* acromion. (From Kock et al. 1996)

If the AC joint width measured on the injured side is placed in the numerator and the value measured on the uninjured side in the denominator, the resulting quotient gives the so-called AC joint index [3].

- A thus determined AC joint index of 1.0 (0.96–1.07; SD 0.03; $p < 0.0001$) is equivalent to a Tossy type I injury.
- An AC joint index of 0.49 (0.31–0.78; SD 0.18; $p < 0.0001$) determined by ultrasound in this manner is equivalent to a Tossy type II instability.
- An ultrasound AC index of 0.21 (0.13–0.24; SD 0.36; $p < 0.0001$) is equivalent to a Tossy type III injury (Figs. 5.1, 5.2, 5.3, and 5.4).

5.5.2 Diagnosis

In the view of the users to date and in the relevant literature on the topic, with sufficient routine the assessment of AC instability in the vertical plane is an easily learned and reliable method. However, in the case of unclear findings (particularly with regard to horizontal instability of the AC joint in terms of Rockwood-IV instability) and other abnormalities, even the experienced surgeon should not hesitate to obtain definitive clarification by means of further imaging (CT and/or MRI).

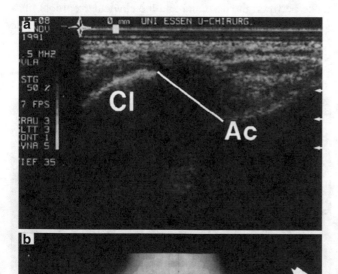

Fig. 5.3 (a) Acromioclavicular joint sonography in a patient with a Tossy II injury on the left (7.5 MHz linear transducer). The sonographically measured AC joint width is left (=injured side) 18 mm and on the right (=non-injured side) 6 mm. Calculated from this the so-called AC joint index is 0.33 (=width of the uninjured side/width of the injured side). (b) Conventional panoramic image of the same patient. *Cl* clavicle, *Ac* acromion. (From Kock et al. 1996)

The extent to which a surgical indication based on exclusively ultrasound evaluation of AC instability can be regarded as the diagnostic standard should be decided by the professional associations as part of the discussions on guidelines for the treatment of acromioclavicular joint instability. Based on the literature on this topic to date, this can only be recommended.

5.5.3 Treatment and Follow-up

In the context of clinical and scientific studies of patients with conservatively or surgically treated AC instability, AC joint ultrasonography appears to be a simple, inexpensive, and informative method without the disadvantage of the radiation exposure associated with X-rays. Therefore, wide-scale application of this method for the purpose of monitoring and follow-up can be recommended without reservation.

5.6 Pitfalls and Red Flags

5.6.1 Horizontal Instability

If there is a clinical suspicion of horizontal acromioclavicular instability, ultrasound is no longer sufficient for exact assessment and radiographic imaging is required.

5.6.2 Accompanying Fracture

Fractures of the ribs, clavicle, and proximal humerus must be excluded. If this is cannot be done with certainty by clinical and ultrasound examination, radiographic imaging is also necessary here.

5.6.3 Epiphyseal Injuries

No valid data are available on epiphyseal injuries. Therefore, an X-ray should be carried out if this injury is suspected.

So far, there is still no international gold standard for the diagnostic imaging of AC joint injuries, neither by ultrasound nor by the radiographic imaging that has been carried out for many decades.

Nevertheless, there is broad agreement that, after the definite exclusion of bony injuries by means of corresponding X-rays, ultrasound examination of AC joint injuries according to the Tossy classification is a suitable and reliable method for making a sufficiently specific diagnosis with regard to the degree of instability of AC joint injuries in terms of vertical instability.

Until the development of a standardized protocol for imaging of AC joint injuries by ultrasound alone, also according to the Rockwood classification (both in the vertical and horizontal plane), X-ray examination particularly for evaluation of horizontal instability and, if necessary, reliable clarification by CT or MRI should be performed.

References

1. Fenkl R, Gotzen L. Die sonografische Diagnostik beim verletzten Akromioklavikulargelenk. Unfallchirurg. 1992;95:393–400.
2. Harland U, Sattler H. Ultraschallfibel Orthopädie, Traumatologie, Rheumatologie. Tokyo: Springer; 1991. p. 50.
3. Kock H-J, Jürgens C, Hirche H, Hanke J, Schmit-Neuerburg K-P. Standardized ultrasound examination for evaluation of instability of the acromioclavicular joint. Arch Orthop Trauma Surg. 1996;115:136–40.
4. Loew M, Sadeghian D, Axhausen K. Sonografische Diagnostik der frischen und veralteten Schultereckgelenksprengung. Orthop Mitt. 1991;3:148.
5. Schmid A, Schmid F. Einsatz der Arthrosonografie bei der Diagnostik von Tossy-Verletzungen am Schultereckgelenk. Aktuelle Traumatol. 1988;18:134–8.
6. Pogorzelski J, Beitzel K, Ranucciu F, Wörtler K, Imhoff AB, Millett PJ, Braun S. The acutely injured acromioclavicular joint—which imaging modalities should be used for accurate diagnosis? A systematic review. BMC Musculoskelet Disord. 2017;18:515–26.
7. Tauber M, Koller H, Hitzl W, Resch H. Dynamic radiologic evaluation of horizontal instability in acute acromioclavicular joint dislocations. Am J Sports Med. 2010;38:1188–95.
8. Ferri M, Finlay K, Popowich T, Jurriaans E, Friedman L. Sonographic examination of the acromioclavicular and sternoclavicular joints. J Clin Ultrasound. 2005;33:345–55.
9. Lee MH, Sheehan SE, Orwin JF, Lee KS. Comprehensive shoulder US examination: a standardized approach with multimodality correlation for common shoulder disease. Radiographics. 2016;36:1606–27.
10. Schneider MM, Balke M, Koenen P, Fröhlich M, Wafaisade A, Bouillon B, Banerjee M. Inter- and intraobserver reliability of the Rockwood classification in acute acromioclavicular joint dislocations. Knee Surg Sports Traumatol Arthrose. 2016;24:2192–6.
11. Tauber M, Hedtmann A, Fett H. Erkrankungen und Verletzungen des Akromio- und Sternoklaviculargelenkes. In: Habermeyer P, et al., editors. Schulterchirurgie. 5. Auflage München: Urban und Fischer Elsevier; 2017. p. S. 287 ff.
12. Vaisman A, Montenegro IEV, De Diego MJT, Ronco JV. A novel radiographic Index for the diagnosis of posterior acromioclavicular joint dislocations. Am J Sports Med. 2014;42:112–6.

Proximal Humerus

Ole Ackermann

6.1 Synopsis

1.1 Rationale of application: fracture diagnosis and determination of the axis deviation of proximal upper arm fractures.

1.2 Evidence level: IIa.

1.3 Indication V.a. proximal upper arm fracture.

1.4 Age of the patient: 0–12 years.

1.5 Examination: Longitudinal section in four levels: Proximal humerus from ventral, lateral, and dorsal in a relieving position; in neutral position humerus from ventral.

1.6 Indications for additional X-ray diagnostics:
  – proven fracture (one plane, exclusion of pathological fracture).
  – persistent pain after 5 days if no fracture has been demonstrated.
  – planned surgery.
  – uncertainty in the assessment.
  – refractures.
  – known bone cyst.
  – no adequate trauma.

1.7 Pitfalls:
  – overlooked clavicle/scapula fracture.
  – pathological fractures (bone cyst, malignant tumor).
  – systemic diseases (i.e., osteogenesis imperfecta).

1.8 Red flags:
  – Fracture without adequate trauma.
  – pre-traumatic complaints at this location.
  – refracture.
  – increasing complaints under therapy.
  – family history of relevant systemic diseases.

1.9 Algorithm: Shoulder SAFE.

O. Ackermann (✉)
Department of Orthopedic Surgery, Ruhr-University Bochum, Bochum, Germany

6.2 Introduction

The proximal humeral fracture (subcapital humeral fracture) in children is significantly less common than the clavicular fracture. Due to the large correction potential at this point, which allows a complete offset of the fragments up to the age of 10 and an axis deviation of up to 40° by the age of 12, and the good representation of the bone, the diagnosis is reliable at this point (Fig. 6.1).

For a long time, the proximal humerus was not the subject of sonographic diagnostics until the problem of measuring an axis deviation was published. This region has certainly benefited from research on the wrist, but ultrasound has also proven to be superior to direct X-ray imaging.

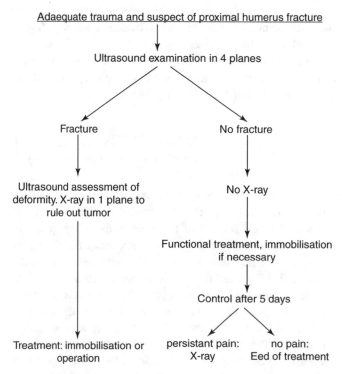

Fig. 6.1 Shoulder SAFE algorithm. (©Ole Ackermann 2020. All rights reserved)

© Springer Nature Switzerland AG 2021
O. Ackermann (ed.), *Fracture Sonography*, https://doi.org/10.1007/978-3-030-63839-9_6

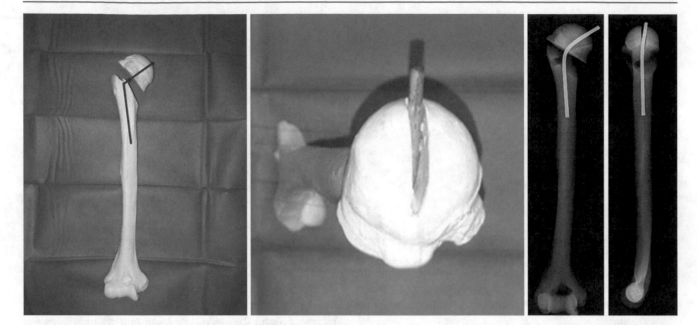

Fig. 6.2 Upper arm phantom; from left to right: clinical phantom from ventral, Clinical phantom from cranial, X-ray phantom strictly a.p., X-ray phantom from the side. (©Ackermann and Eckert 2015; Courtesy of off label media)

The surgical indication for this injury is based on the axis deviation. However, the X-ray does not provide a clear picture of the position in which the bone was X-rayed and whether there are really two planes that are perpendicular to each other. Such an assessment is very difficult even in adults, but even more in children with not fully developed bony landmarks. Experience shows that small patients are not sufficiently compliant due to the existing pain to allow correct X-ray projections. But then the measurement of the axis deviation, although highly relevant for the therapy decision, is only a rough estimate.

The projection error occurs due to deviations in the rotation and tilt of the bone in relation to the image plane and can be quantified using the following formula:

$$\alpha' = \arccos\left(\frac{\cos\alpha\cos\beta + \sin\alpha\sin\beta\sin\rho}{\sqrt{\left(\sin\alpha\cos\rho\right)^2 + \left(\cos\alpha\cos\beta + \sin\alpha\sin\beta\sin\rho\right)^2}}\right)$$

α' = optical deviation of the bone in the image plane (analogous to the X-ray image); α = actual deviation of the fragment in degrees; β = tilt of the bone to the image plane in degrees (analogous to the ante- and retroversion on the upper arm); ρ = rotation of the bone in degrees (analogous to the inner and outer rotation on the upper arm). arccos = arc cosine, sin = sine, cos = cosine. All angles in degrees. (Derivation from Prof. Marc Levine, Essen; see literature)

Even if the representation is correct, the axis deviation of the fracture is almost never depicted orthogradally, because the direction of the axis deviation is not exactly in one of the two planes shown. If, in the case of a 40° axis deviation, this is rotated by 45°, the result is an incorrect measurement of 9.3° (23%), i.e., a span of 31.7–49.3°; there is therefore a relevant potential for misjudgments, which until now was only of minor clinical importance due

to the high correction potential. Nevertheless, a better measurement is desirable.

This example is illustrated below (Fig. 6.2):

Here a wire bent in the frontal plane 120° in an upper arm phantom a.p. and X-rayed on the side and displayed correctly. If, however, the wire is rotated ventrally by 45°, the X-ray examination shows a false–low bend of the wire despite correctly set planes (which in reality corresponds to an axis deviation estimated as wrong–low) (Fig. 6.3).

Fracture sonography offers a solution here. Not only can fractures be diagnosed or excluded, but the deformation can also be displayed with high precision. The reason for this is that the bone is assessed from four projections and any other levels can be displayed. In a sectional plane parallel to the bone axis, an axis deviation can be underestimated but not overestimated, so that the image plane with the maximum axis deviation is always searched for and used for the measurement.

A disadvantage of fracture sonography is that it cannot display intraosseous processes and therefore does not detect bone cysts and tumors, which are not uncommon at this point. For this reason, if a fracture is proven, an X-ray image in one plane is always necessary to exclude a pathological fracture (Fig. 6.4).

The main benefit of fracture sonography at this point is the exclusion of fractures and the determination of the axis in the case of bony injuries.

6.3 Indication Including Patient Age

In patients from 0 to 12 years of age, primary fracture diagnosis can be carried out at this point based on ultrasound. The accident mechanism is a fall or impact on the shoulder. Fractures of the clavicle (common) and the scapula/acro-

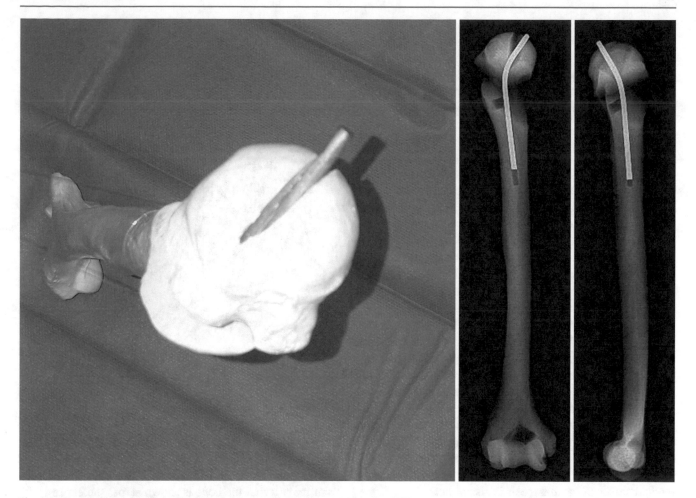

Fig. 6.3 From left to right: clinically oblique phantom; X-ray phantom a.p., rotated 10°; X-ray phantom rotated 10° to the side. (©Ackermann and Eckert 2015; Courtesy of off label media)

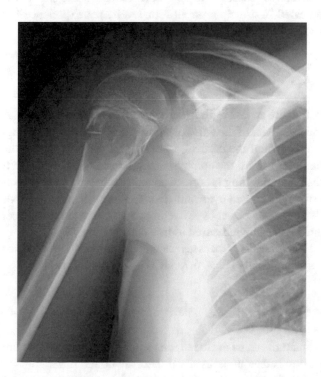

Fig. 6.4 X-ray pathological proximal humeral fracture in a bone cyst. (©Ackermann and Eckert 2015; Courtesy of off label media)

mion (very rare) and shoulder dislocation (extremely rare) must and can be excluded by palpation.

If there is no adequate accident mechanism, a pathological fracture is likely and full radiological imaging is mandatory.

Local pain is indicated during the physical examination, and mobility is usually significantly restricted. Bead, kink, and epiphyseal injuries (mostly type Aitken I) occur.

Fracture sonography should be avoided if there is already a clinically clear deformity and a safe surgical indication. The representation of highly dislocated fragments is difficult and has no therapeutic benefit.

6.4 Contraindications and Indications for X-ray Diagnostics

If a vascular or nerve injury is suspected, sonography should not be carried out, since complex injuries are to be expected here and rapid further radiological diagnostics, including sectional imaging, must be carried out. The additional benefit of sonography is limited here, so we do not recommend using it in these cases.

If a clear surgical indication is already given during the clinical examination, sonography is superfluous. At the current point in time, we recommend preoperative X-ray diagnostics for planning the procedure for all planned operations so that one of the rare complex damage patterns (e.g., multi-fragmentary zones) is not overlooked. This also applies if the surgical indication is only made sonographically.

If the finding cannot be reliably assessed, the diagnosis can be verified by displaying different levels (see examination). If there is still no clarity, an X-ray examination is indicated. This is usually the case at the beginning of the application of fracture sonography and is rarely necessary for the experienced examiner. However, it is better to make your own diagnosis and to take an additional X-ray picture than to delay the process with repeated checks and to unsettle therapists and patients with unsafe diagnostics. Such an X-ray check also serves to confirm your own sonographic diagnosis and thus to gain certainty in the assessment of findings.

If no fracture is primarily diagnosed sonographically, an X-ray check should be carried out after 5 days if symptoms persist. A renewed sonography will show no result other than the primary examination and is therefore unnecessary. In such a case, the clavicle and scapula including the acromion and AC joint should be examined again.

If there is no adequate trauma, in the case of refractures and pre-traumatic symptoms, X-ray diagnostics should be carried out to rule out pathological processes such as bone cysts and tumors. If there is a family history for relevant systemic diseases, X-ray diagnosis is also indicated.

6.4.1 Investigation

Diagnostics and therapy follow the Shoulder SAFE algorithm.

After taking the medical history and the clinical examination, the sonographic examination follows.

6.4.2 Positioning

The little patient sits on the examination couch, next to or on the lap of the parents. The arm is usually held spontaneously in a relieving position with the forearm on, so that the examination begins in this position.

6.4.3 Levels

Three longitudinal sections from ventral, lateral, and dorsal are shown in a careful posture. The forearm is then carefully turned to the neutral position, 90° to the body axis, and the fourth longitudinal section is shown from the ventral side. If a fracture appears, the projection with the greatest axis deviation can be displayed and documented by moving around the humeral head (Figs. 6.5 and 6.6).

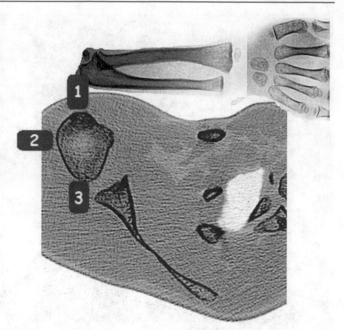

Fig. 6.5 Sonographic levels 1–3. (©Ackermann and Eckert 2015; Courtesy of off label media)

6.4.4 Examination Procedure

Finding the bone is no problem. After showing the bone, which is shown as a bright, sharp line, the transducer is first aligned parallel to the longitudinal axis. This can be seen from the fact that the bone is shown across the entire width of the image section. Then the epiphyseal plate is shown. The correct setting has now been reached. The process is repeated in principle on all four levels, but experience has shown that this is very easy after the first setting.

6.4.5 Evaluation

A fracture appears as a kink, bulge, offset, or fracture gap. A measurement of the axis deviation is based on the physiological course of the cortical, whereby here the bending of the humerus toward the epiphysis must be taken into account. If the parallel setting is correct, an axis deviation can be underestimated, but not overestimated. Therefore, the greatest axis deviation can be set by swiveling and moving the transducer and this can be measured as true deformation.

Intraosseous processes cannot be adequately assessed sonographically (Figs. 6.7, 6.8, 6.9, 6.10, and 6.11).

6.4.6 Diagnosis

A fracture can be excluded sonographically. An X-ray examination is then unnecessary if there are no red flags.

If a fracture is detected, an X-ray is always taken on one level, regardless of the indication for surgery, in order to

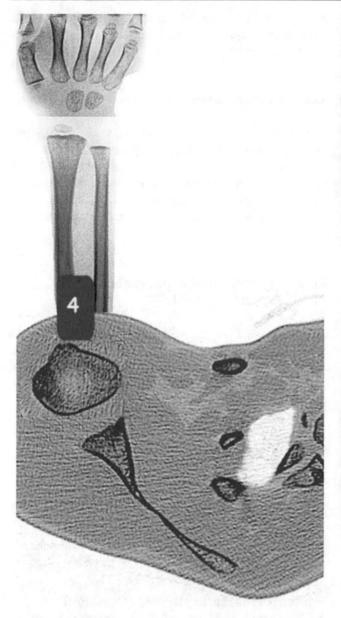

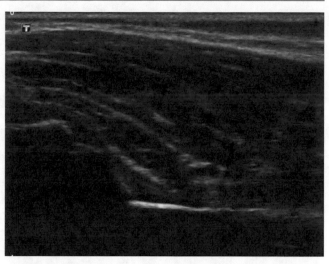

Fig. 6.8 Upper arm fracture shapes: Knick. (©Ackermann and Eckert 2015; Courtesy of off label media)

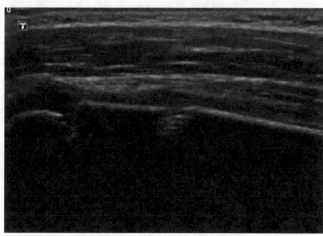

Fig. 6.9 Upper am fracture forms: gap. (©Ackermann and Eckert 2015; Courtesy of off label media)

Fig. 6.6 Sonographic levels 2. (©Ackermann and Eckert 2015; Courtesy of off label media)

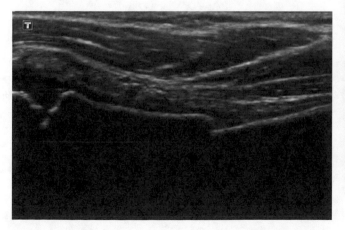

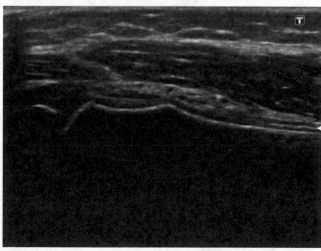

Fig. 6.10 Fracture shapes on the upper arm: bulge. (©Ackermann and Eckert 2015; Courtesy of off label media)

Fig. 6.7 Upper am fracture forms: offset. (©Ackermann and Eckert 2015; Courtesy of off label media)

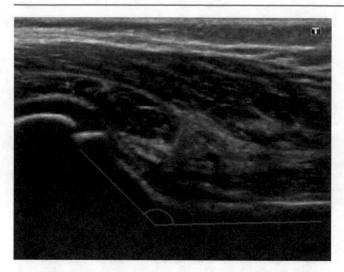

Fig. 6.11 Axial deviation measurement of upper arm. (©Ackermann and Eckert 2015; Courtesy of off label media)

identify pathological fractures. This automatically includes the admission to surgery planning. In the standard procedure, an operation indication is made based on the axis deviation measured sonographically.

Radiological clarification is also carried out if other osseous pathologies such as an osteitis, cyst, or the like are suspected.

With all uncertainties in the diagnosis, the additional X-ray examination is permitted.

6.5 Therapy and Controls

The therapy is based on the generally known guidelines for proximal upper arm fracture in growing age. The pain-adapted immobilization in a Gilchrist bandage if the indication is conservative. We only perform sonographic position checks if there is evidence of a dislocation clinically (inspectorally or due to increased pain), which is rarely the case. A sonographic consolidation check is also not mandatory if there is no clinical palpation pain.

If no fracture is diagnosed sonographically, the therapy is pain-adapted. Functional treatment is given for only discrete complaints, and immobilization occurs if there is significant pain. All of these patients are checked on the fifth day after the accident. If there is still palpation pain or swelling at this point, an X-ray check is carried out on two levels; if the result is bland, the therapy is completed.

6.6 Pitfalls and Red Flags

6.6.1 Pathological Fracture

A pathological fracture must not be overlooked due to the therapeutic consequences. Since this cannot be reliably represented sonographically, an X-ray check is carried out on one level for all detected fractures. According to the authors, a large enough cyst to provoke a fracture can always be represented on one level.

6.6.2 Systemic Diseases

Broken bones or refractions without adequate trauma, previous operations with a septic component, signs of inflammation, or pre-traumatic symptoms as well as a family history indicate a deeper or systemic disease and should be clarified radiologically. Sonography always shows only the bone surface and the pathologies that can be identified there.

6.6.3 Increasing Pain/Spontaneous Expression of Pain

If the symptoms increase with adequate therapy or if the child spontaneously reports pain in the Gilchrist, precise clinical control is mandatory. Instability should be excluded by palpatory imaging and fractures of other bones (clavicle, scapula, acromion).

Further Reading

Formula for the Projection of the Axis Deviation

1. Ackermann O, Levine M, Eckert K, Rülander C, Stanjek M, Schulze-Pellengahr C. Unsicherheit bei der radiologischen Achsbestimmung proximaler Humerusfrakturen. Z Orthop Unfall. 2013;151:74–9.

Problem of Measuring the Axis Deviation in the X-ray Image, Superiority of Sonography to X-ray Imaging when Measuring the Axis Deviation

2. Ackermann O, Sesia S, Berberich T, Liedgens P, Eckert K, Großer K, Roessler M, Rülander C, Vogel T. Sonographische Diagnostik der subcapitalen Humerusfraktur im Wachstumsalter. Der Unfallchirurg. 2010;113:839–44.

Shoulder SAFE

3. Eckert K, Ackermann O. Sonographische Frakturdiagnostik. Der Radiologe. 2015;55:992–9.

Screening for Elbow Fractures

Kolja Eckert

7.1 Synopsis

1.1 Indication: Primary sonographic evaluation of child-hood elbow injuries.

1.2 Rationale of use: Exclusion of a fracture close to the elbow by diagnosis of the intra-articular effusion; the actual fracture diagnosis with positive fat pad signs is always done radiologically.

1.3 Evidence level: IIá.

1.4 Contraindications: open injuries, clinically safe vascular or nerve damage, clearly visible malposition with clinically safe surgical indication, insufficient patient compliance.

1.5 Age of the patient: 0–12 years.

1.6 Examination: medical history, clinical examination, ultrasound: longitudinal median section over the fossa olecrani.

1.7 Indications for additional X-ray diagnostics:
   – sonographically positive fat pad sign (SOnographic FAt pad sign (SOFA⊕)).
   – Persistent pain or swelling after 5–7 days, even if there was no evidence of a fracture initially with ultrasound.
   – safe surgical indication.
   – uncertainty in the assessment.
   – refractures.

1.8 Pitfalls:
   – Ulnar epicondyle fractures (eventually no effusion).
   – Radial head torus fractures (eventually no effusion).
   – Humeral or forearm shaft fractures near the joint (no effusion).
   – Pathological fractures (e.g. osteogenesis imperfecta, bone cysts).

1.9 Red flags:
   – severe pain/immobility even without a sonographic fracture indication.
   – no adequate trauma.

   – pre-traumatic complaints at this location.
   – refracture.
   – increasing complaints under therapy.
   – persistent elbow pain under therapy.

1.10 Algorithm:
   – Elbow SAFE (see Fig. 7.1).

7.2 Introduction

Elbow injuries are a common injury in pediatric and trauma emergency rooms and practices. A X-ray examination of the affected elbow in two planes has so far been the gold standard in fracture diagnostics and is used frequently and generously. X-ray diagnostics should be used specifically to detect a fracture. Clinical experience shows, however, that the number of fractures discovered with the X-ray is small, so that in the sense of radiation hygiene it is sensible to establish alternative and radiation-free imaging even in the case of elbow injuries.

With three joint-forming bones, the elbow joint offers a wide range of different fractures and thus a diagnostic and therapeutic challenge. The cartilaginous humeral epiphysis with its different age-related bone cores can also make a reliable diagnosis of a fracture difficult on an X-ray.

The growth joints of the elbow only make up about 20% of the length of the arm. Therefore, there is only a small correction potential for displaced elbow fractures and the demands on diagnostics and therapy are particularly high. In addition to the correct fracture diagnosis, the imaging procedure must also enable a reliable assessment of a malposition.

The most common fracture at the child's elbow joint is the supracondylar humeral fracture followed by the radial condyle fracture and the ulnar epicondyle. Other, less common fractures are olecranon fractures and radius neck fractures. The accident mechanism for an elbow joint fracture is typically falling on the outstretched arm or, less often, on the bent elbow. A direct impact trauma to the elbow is very painful due to the thin soft tissue covering, but a fracture is rather unlikely.

K. Eckert (✉)
Marienhospital Gelsenkirchen, Klinik für Kinderchirurgie, Gelsenkirchen, Germany

Fig. 7.1 Elbow-SAFE (sonographic algorithm for fracture evaluation). (©Ole Ackermann 2020. All rights reserved)

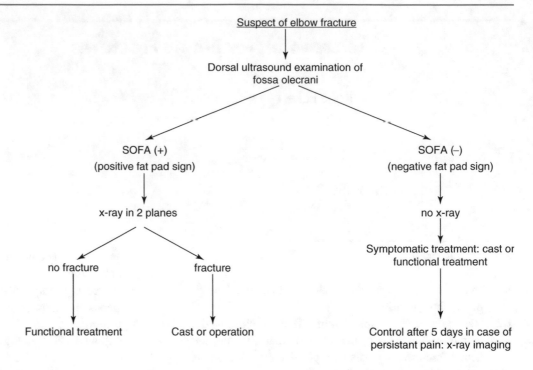

Basically, a child traumatologist and sonographically experienced examiner can also diagnose and classify all fractures of the child's elbow joint sonographically as such. However, in comparison to other skeletal sections, a comprehensive sonographic representation of the elbow joint is time-consuming. On the one hand, this requires at least nine standard cuts, which are not always easy to adjust in the event of an injury. On the other hand, the ultrasound examination can be very painful for the children, especially if a fracture is present. A complete and diagnostically reliable sonographic examination of an elbow fracture is therefore only possible to a limited extent even for the experienced examiner.

Nevertheless, ultrasound can also be used sensibly in the case of childhood elbow injuries. Every intra-articular elbow joint fracture leads to a more or less pronounced joint effusion and thus to a lifting of the rear fat pad from the fossa olecrani. Norell [1] and Bledsoe and Izenstark [2] were able to show that a liftoff of the posterior fat pad can be shown in the lateral X-ray image of the elbow and thus indicates a fracture as a so-called positive fat pad sign even without a direct fracture sign.

As early as [3], Miles was able to show that a positive posterior fat pad sign as a typical soft tissue lesion can also be detected very sensitively using sonography. With a sensitivity of 97% and a specificity of 90%, a sonographically positive or negative posterior fat pad sign can detect or rule out an elbow joint fracture [4, 5]. This makes the sonographic fat pad sign (SOnographic FAt pad sign (SOFA)) an ideal screening parameter in the primary evaluation of childhood elbow injuries.

The sonographic examination to detect or exclude a posterior fat pad sign can be carried out in less than a minute and is painless. After only a little practice, even those with little experience in ultrasound diagnostics can make a reliable assessment.

Elbow injuries that occur frequently and for which no fracture is predominantly found are therefore the ideal indication for ultrasound, so that numerous X-ray examinations can be saved.

Due to the increased use of ultrasound, additional waiting times in the X-ray department are eliminated, so that the overall examination time is shortened.

7.3 Indications

The particular benefit of sonography is the primary evaluation of childhood elbow injuries in order to detect or rule out fractures qualitatively in terms of screening, using the sonographic fat pad sign (SOnographic FAt pad sign (SOFA)).

For the reason that with a sonographically positive dorsal fat pad sign (SOFA⊕) an intra-articular elbow joint fracture is likely, an additional X-ray examination of the elbow is indicated. With a negative fat pad sign (SOFA⊖), however, a fracture of the elbow joint is very unlikely and an additional X-ray examination can be dispensed for the time being.

7.4 Contraindications to Ultrasound Diagnostics

Especially in the case of an obvious malposition and thus a clinically clear indication for surgery, sonography is not useful and can at most be an additional burden for the child.

Preoperative X-ray diagnostics are mandatory for planning surgery and procedures.

In the case of open injuries (e.g., grazes) of the elbow, primary sonography is not contraindicated, but should be used carefully to avoid possible wound infection and unnecessary pain.

Since there is still insufficient experience for ultrasound screening after previous operations or fractures on the elbow, its use in these cases is currently possible, but is not yet fully recommended.

If the clinical examination indicates an additional vascular or nerve injury, duplex sonography of the vessels can be useful in addition to the sonographic fat pad mark and provide advice that is crucial for therapy. However, since complex injuries are to be expected here, an ultrasound examination should not delay targeted diagnosis and therapy.

If the sonographic assessment of a positive fat pad sign (SOFA⊕) is uncertain or unclear, an examination of the opposite side can be helpful. If there is still uncertainty then, as with all uncertainties, an X-ray examination should be carried out.

7.5 Examination

An exact medical history and the most precise clinical examination possible are essential for every indication for imaging.

In addition to soft tissue swelling and localized pressure pain (radial condyle, epicondyle ulnaris, on the olecranon or radial head), the clinical examination should also take into account pain during the turning movement or restricted flexion/extension due to pain.

Furthermore, fractures of the humeral or forearm shaft close to the joint must be clinically excluded.

After taking the medical history and the clinical examination, the sonographic examination is immediately carried out by the same examiner, ideally without changing the examination room.

7.5.1 Positioning

The sonographic screening examination on the elbow (dorsomedian longitudinal section above the fossa olecrani) makes no special demands on the patient positioning. Experience shows that most patients keep the affected elbow in a slightly flexed position. The dorsal elbow region is thus easily accessible for ultrasound examination of the injured arm after the sleeve has been pulled up (Fig. 7.2). The child can sit or lie on a chair or an examination couch at his or her convenience, next to or on the parents' lap. It is also generally not necessary to darken the room.

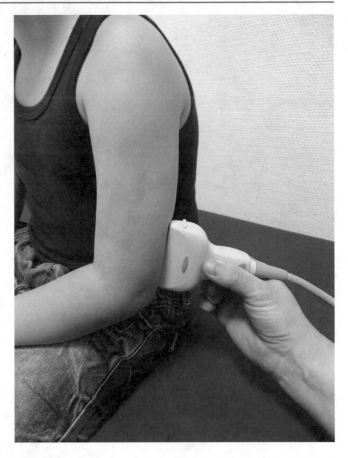

Fig. 7.2 The linear transducer is placed on the elbow from the dorsal side. The child can be seated on a chair or an examination couch or lying down, next to or on the parents' lap. (©Ackermann and Eckert 2015; Courtesy of off label media)

7.5.2 Levels

The ultrasound screening on the elbow with the median longitudinal section above the fossa olecrani (Fig. 7.3) only requires one projection. Even the inexperienced examiner can quickly display the fossa olecrani. Using the criteria shown below (see below), an effusion of the joint can be quickly identified, a distinction made between a negative and a positive dorsal fat pad sign (SOFA⊕/SOFA⊖), and the presence of an elbow joint fracture can thus be estimated.

7.5.3 Evaluation

The so-called dorsal fat pad has an intra-articular and extra-synovial position and is located in the fossa olecrani (Fig. 7.4). An intra-articular elbow joint fracture always leads to more or less joint effusion, which lifts the fat pad dorsally out of its position from the olecranon fossa (Fig. 7.5). The effusion and fat pad can then be seen in the exactly lateral X-ray image of the elbow.

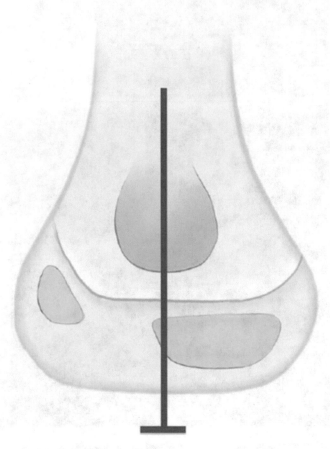

Fig. 7.3 Dorsomedian longitudinal section over the fossa olecrani. (©Ackermann and Eckert 2015; Courtesy of off label media)

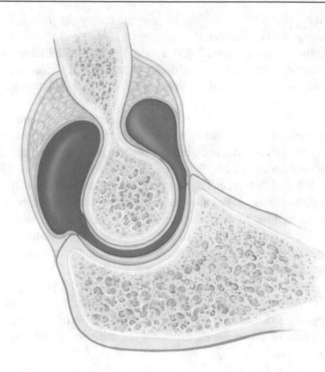

Fig. 7.5 In the case of an elbow effusion, the ventral and dorsal fat pad are each convexly arched out of the coronoid and olecrani fossa

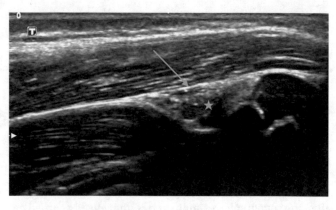

Fig. 7.6 Elbow flexion: without effusion of the joint, the dorsal fat pad (asterisk) lies in the olecrani fossa. The joint capsule (arrow) attaches to the dorsal humeral cortex at an acute angle. (©Ackermann and Eckert 2014; Courtesy of off label media)

As a typical soft tissue lesion, an articular effusion with the raised dorsal fat pad can be shown very sensitively using ultrasound.

Without effusion of the joint, i.e., with negative fat pad signs (SOFA⊖), there is always an acute-angled attachment of the elbow joint capsule to the dorsal humeral cortex. In the case of elbow flexion, the joint capsule extends as an echo-rich line in a straight line from the dorsal humeral cortex (Fig. 7.6). When the elbow is extended, the dorsal joint capsule shows a dorsally concave configuration (Fig. 7.7). Only with complete extension can the representation of the fossa olecrani be difficult due to an overlay by the olecranon. Clinical experience shows, however, that the affected elbow

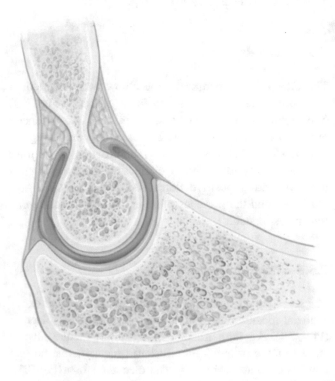

Fig. 7.4 The dorsal fat pad (yellow) has an intracapsular (red) but extrasynovial (green) position

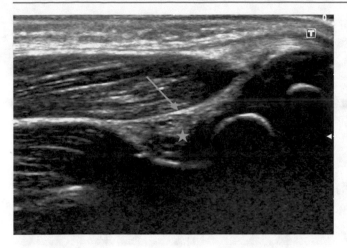

Fig. 7.7 Elbow extension: the dorsal fat pad (star) remains in the fossa olecrani. The joint capsule (arrow) is still attached to the dorsal humeral cortex at an acute angle. (©Ackermann and Eckert 2014; Courtesy of off label media)

mostly cannot be stretched if the fracture is actually present and that the children hold the arm in a flexion position.

In the case of an intra-articular elbow joint fracture, the effusion lifts the fat pad out of the olecrani fossa and bulges the joint capsule in a dorsally convex curve (Figs. 7.8 and 7.9). In addition, at the base of the dorsal humeral cortex, the capsule may be raised to the dorso-cranial direction (Figs. 7.10 and 7.11). Even small amounts of effusion can be detected very sensitively. An echo-rich effusion, possibly with mirror formation, indicates hemarthrosis and a fracture is therefore obvious (Figs. 7.12 and 7.13).

7.5.4 Diagnosis

All elbow fractures are accompanied by a sonographically verifiable effusion. The ultrasound can qualitatively detect or exclude a fracture based on the dorsal fat pad sign. An addi-

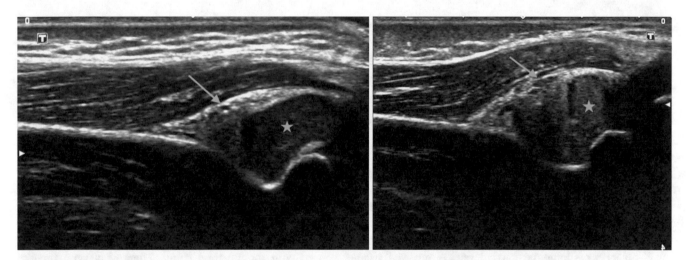

Figs. 7.8 and 7.9 In the case of a joint effusion (asterisk), the joint capsule (arrow) bulges convexly dorsally. (©Ackermann and Eckert 2014; Courtesy of off label media)

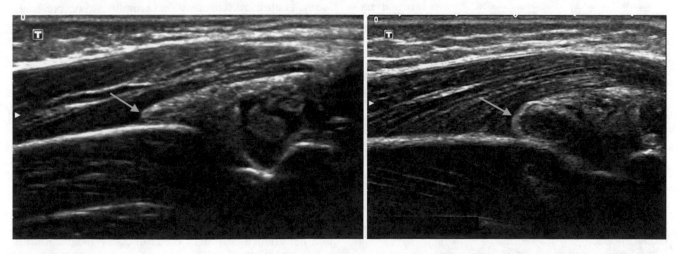

Figs. 7.10 and 7.11 With a positive fat pad sign, in some cases, there is also a bulge (arrow) of the joint capsule on the dorsal humeral cortex. (©Ackermann and Eckert 2014, 2015; Courtesy of off label media)

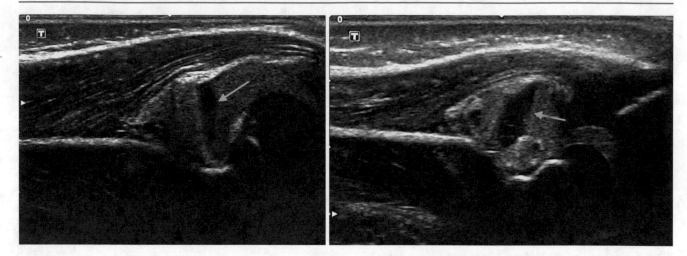

Figs. 7.12 and 7.13 An echo-rich joint effusion with mirror formation (arrow) indicates a hemarthrosis and thus a safe existing elbow joint fracture. The ultrasound image is tilted by 90° in relation to the arm posture during examination, so that the mirror formation comes perpendicular to the display. (©Ackermann and Eckert 2014, 2015; Courtesy of off label media)

tional X-ray examination is always necessary for an accurate diagnosis of fractures.

The value of ultrasound screening on the elbow is to exclude a fracture sonographically so that an X-ray examination is not necessary for these patients.

7.5.5 Therapy and Controls

If initially there is no clinical or sonographic (SOFA⊖) evidence of a fracture, symptom-oriented treatment is carried out, which can be carried out functionally in the case of moderate complaints, or with cast immobilization in the case of more severe complaints. If symptoms persist for 7 days, an X-ray check should be carried out. A renewed sonographic examination gives no other result than the primary examination and is therefore unnecessary.

In the case of sonographically positive fat pad signs (SOFA⊕), a standard X-ray examination of the elbow is carried out, since a fracture is likely.

7.6 Elbow-SAFE

A reliable diagnosis and therapy can only be achieved by looking at the medical history, clinical, and imaging findings. From this, an algorithm was developed that enables a safe and widely radiation-free diagnosis of childhood elbow injuries. In the sonographic algorithm for fracture evaluation on the elbow (Elbow-SAFE), the sonographic fat pad sign is used as a screening parameter in the primary evaluation of elbow injuries.

The Elbow-SAFE (Fig. 7.1) is applicable for children up to 12 years of age and is based on a precise medical history

(adequate trauma?), a clinical examination, and then on a focused ultrasound examination (median longitudinal section above the fossa olecrani) on the elbow to be able to distinguish between a negative or positive dorsal fat sign (SOFA⊕ or SOFA⊖?).

In the case of sonographically positive fat pad signs (SOFA⊕), a standard X-ray examination of the elbow is carried out in two projections in order to detect and precisely diagnose a fracture. The therapy is based on the X-ray diagnosis and is carried out in accordance with the standard of traumatology for children.

In the case of sonographically negative fat pad signs (SOFA⊖), an intra-articular elbow joint fracture is very unlikely and an additional X-ray examination can be dispensed with for the time being. Therapy is symptomatic. However, the patients should be symptom-free or at least significantly less symptom-free after about 7 days, otherwise an X-ray control is indicated for progressive or persistent complaints.

7.7 Pitfalls and Red Flags

A sonographically positive fat pad sign only allows a qualitative statement about the high probability of an elbow joint fracture.

Humeral or forearm shaft fractures near the elbow joint must be clinically assessed through a subtle medical history and clinical examination. If there is suspicion, the transducer can be guided proximally or distally over the upper and lower arm to search for a fracture. Nevertheless, if there is clinical suspicion, but also in the case of sonographic fracture detection in the shaft area, an X-ray examination is recommended to ensure a reliable estimate of the axis deviation.

Since the ulnar epicondyle is only partially intra-articular, corresponding fractures can only lead to a slight formation of effusion, so that a fracture can be underestimated, especially initially and especially with only a slight dislocation. Therefore, if there is any clinical suspicion (pressure pain, swelling over the ulnar epicondyle), an additional X-ray examination is indicated.

Even with metaphyseal bead fractures of the proximal radius, due to the minimal trauma, only a small amount of effusion and therefore possibly no sonographically detectable fat pad signs are possible. However, since these fractures cannot always be reliably diagnosed radiologically, and conservative therapy using Cast immobilization is indicated both in the case of a proven fracture and in the case of clinical suspicion alone, there is no other therapeutic consequence even with sonographically negative fat pad signs.

Since sonography does not allow an assessment of intraosseous processes, X-ray diagnostics should also be carried out in the event of refractures or inadequate trauma in order to rule out pathological processes (cysts, osteomyelitis, foreign bodies, bone malformation, or healing disorders).

Radius-head subluxation (Chaissagnac lesion) is a clinical diagnosis in childhood and usually requires no additional imaging. Ultrasound screening can only be helpful if the patient's anamnesis is unclear, in order to be able to reliably identify a fracture based on a positive fat pad sign or to attempt a reduction if the fat pad sign is negative.

At the present time, there is insufficient experience with fracture sonography for refractures, which is why X-rays should be taken in case of doubt.

References

Sonographic Fracture Diagnosis on the Child's Elbow

1. Norell HG. Roentgenologic visualization of the extracapsular fat; its importance in the diagnosis of traumatic injuries to the elbow. Acta Radiol. 1954;42:205–10.
2. Bledsoe RC, Izenstark JL. Displacement of fat pads in disease and injury of the elbow: a new radiographic sign. Radiology. 1959;73:717–24.
3. Miles KA, Lamont AC. Ultrasonic demonstration of the elbow fat pads. Clin Radiol. 1989;40:602–4.
4. Eckert K, Ackermann O, Janssen N, et al. Accuracy of the sonographic fat pad sign for primary screening of pediatric elbow fractures: a preliminary study. J Med Ultrason. 2014;41(4):473–80.
5. Rabiner JE, Khine H, Avner JR, et al. Accuracy of point-of-care ultrasonography for diagnosis of elbow fractures in children. Ann Emerg Med. 2013;61:9–17.

Further Reading

6. Eckert K, Ackermann O, Schweiger B, et al. Ultrasound evaluation of elbow fractures in children. J Med Ultrason. 2013;40:443–51.
7. Davidson RS, Markowitz RI, Dormans J, et al. Ultrasonographic evaluation of the elbow in infants and young children after suspected trauma. J Bone Joint Surg Am. 1994;76:1804–13.
8. Grechenig W, Clement HG, Schatz B, et al. Sonographic examination of trauma to the elbow and hand. Orthopade. 2002;31:271–7.
9. Markowitz RI, Davidson RS, Harty MP, et al. Sonography of the elbow in infants and children. AJR. 1992;159:829–33.
10. Martinoli C, Bianchi S, Zamorani MP, et al. Ultrasound of the elbow. Eur J Ultrasound. 2001;14:21–7.
11. Pistor G, Graffstädt H. Sonographic diagnosis of supracondylar fractures of the humerus retrospective and prospective studies in children. Ultraschall Med. 2003;24:331–9.
12. Tran N, Chow K. Ultrasonography of the elbow. Semin Musculoskelet Radiol. 2007;11:105–16.
13. Zhang JD, Chen H. Ultrasonography for non-displaced and mini-displaced humeral lateral condyle fractures in children. Chin J Traumatol. 2008;11:297–300.
14. Zuazo I, Bonnefoy O, Tauzin C, et al. Acute elbow trauma in children: role of ultrasonography. Pediatr Radiol. 2008;38:982–8.

A Positive Posterior Fat Sign Indicates a Fracture

15. Dihlmann SW, Meenen NM, Wolf L, et al. Fettpolsterzeichen und Supinatorfettlinie bei Kubitaltraumen. Unfallchirurgie. 1992;18:148–53.
16. Major NM, Crawford ST. Elbow effusions in trauma in adults and children: is there an occult fracture? AJR. 2002;178:413–8.
17. O'Dwyer H, O'Sullivan P, Fitzgerald D, et al. The fat pad sign following elbow trauma in adults: its usefulness and reliability in suspecting occult fracture. J Comput Assist Tomogr. 2004;28:562–5.
18. Kohn AM. Soft tissue alterations in elbow trauma. Am J Roentgenol. 1959;82:867–74.
19. Vyhánek L, Teisinger P, Eckert V, Druga R. Die Weichteilveränderungen beim Trauma des Ellenbogens und der peripheren Radiusepiphyse. Fortschr Röntgenstr. 1970;112:505–9.
20. Fick DS, Lyons TA. Interpreting elbow radiographs in children. Am Fam Physician. 1997;55:1278–82.
21. Kraus R, Berthold LD, von Laer L. Efficient imaging of elbow injuries in children and adolescents. Klin Padiatr. 2007;219:282–7.
22. Skaggs D, Pershad J. Pediatric elbow trauma. Pediatr Emerg Care. 1997;13:425–34.

A Negative Fat Pad Sign Is Very Likely to Rule Out a Fracture

23. Donnelly LF, Klostermeier TT, Klosterman LA. Traumatic elbow effusions in pediatric patients: are occult fractures the rule? AJR. 1998;171:243–5.

Ultrasound Is more Sensitive to SOFA than X-rays

24. De Maeseneer M, Jacobson JA, Jaovisidha S, et al. Elbow effusions: distribution of joint fluid with flexion and extension and imaging implications. Investig Radiol. 1998;33:117–25.

Distal Forearm

Ole Ackermann

8.1 Synopsis

1.1 Rationale of application: X-ray-free diagnosis and therapy of childhood distal forearm fractures.

1.2 Evidence level: Ia.

1.3 Indication: X-ray-free diagnosis and therapy control if distal forearm fracture is suspected in children.

1.4 Contraindications: open fractures, V.a. Vascular/nerve damage, clearly visible malposition, safe surgical indication.

1.5 Age of the patient: 0–12 years.

1.6 Examination: longitudinal section in six planes: radius from dorsal, radial and volar, ulna from dorsal, ulnar and volar.

1.7 Indications for additional X-ray diagnostics:
- persistent pain after 5 days if no fracture has been demonstrated.
- planned surgery.
- uncertainty in the assessment.
- refractions.
- suspect of carpal/scaphoid fracture (MRI).
- no adequate trauma.

1.8 Pitfalls:
- carpal fractures.
- additional shaft fractures or proximal forearm fractures.
- undisplaced epiphyseal plate injuries.
- systemic diseases (i.e., osteogenesis imperfecta).

1.9 Red flags:
- severe pain/immobility without proof of fracture.
- fracture without adequate trauma.
- pre-traumatic complaints at this location.
- refracture.
- increasing complaints under therapy.

- family history of relevant systemic diseases.
- wrist pain after 5 days.

1.10 Algorithm: Wrist SAFE (Fig. 8.1).

8.2 Introduction

The distal forearm fracture is by far the most common fracture in childhood with about 40% and is treated regularly in every traumatological practice and clinic outpatient clinic. At the same time, this bone fracture is very benign with an enormous correction potential, so that axis deviations of up to 40° can theoretically be left up to the age of 12, since these reliably balance each other out. The disadvantage of clearly visible axis deviations is that a limitation of the rotation is accepted until the axis is corrected, so that we recommend a reduction in our own procedure if the turning movement is mechanically restricted (Fig. 8.1).

The lightly curved bone and the thin soft tissue coat facilitate the sonographic display at this point, so that even beginners in fracture sonography can carry out reliable diagnostics and therapy control here. The frequent occurrence of the injury also ensures a training effect, which guarantees a constant occupation with the topic. The large number of patients also means that many X-ray images can be saved in radiation-sensitive children.

The examination is painless and can be carried out quickly. For the practice, the sonographic examination takes about 1 min.

The sonographic diagnosis of the distal wrist in children is therefore the ideal entry-level indication for beginners in fracture sonography.

Historically, fracture sonography has long been used on a child's wrist, first published by Saphoznikow in 1978. Because of the favorable conditions, the child's wrist was always the favorite child of fracture sonography with the most publications. Ultimately, however, research was limited to demonstrating that the fracture could be visualized sonographically. It was not until 2006 that the systematic com-

O. Ackermann (✉)
Department of Orthopedic Surgery, Ruhr-University Bochum, Bochum, Germany

© Springer Nature Switzerland AG 2021
O. Ackermann (ed.), *Fracture Sonography*, https://doi.org/10.1007/978-3-030-63839-9_8

Fig. 8.1 Wrist SAFE algorithm. (©Ole Ackermann 2020. All rights reserved)

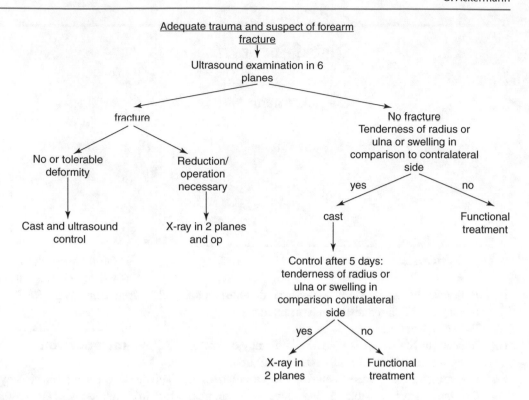

parison with X-ray diagnostics was carried out, which ultimately paved the way for clinical application. The development of a fixed algorithm was another step in this direction. In 2016, the indication was confirmed in a meta study (Douma den Hamer, see literature).

The historical gold standard was X-rays in two planes. Our own studies indicate that the rate of false-negative results in ultrasound diagnostics and X-ray imaging are identical. Small fractures can be masked by the superimposed representation of the bones on the X-ray image, and smaller edge fractures are rarely not shown on the ultrasound. However, due to the large potential for correction, these overlooked findings do not seem to be of medical importance if the treatment is based on findings and if the pain in the plaster cast is immobilized. However, the results show that fracture sonography has the potential to become an alternative gold standard for this pathology.

8.3 Indication

The indication for fracture sonography is the suspicion of a distal forearm fracture in children up to 12 years of age. While children actively point out pain after learning a language, younger children are sparing and expressing displeasure when touching the extremity.

Up to this age, the "childlike" fracture forms appear: bead, kink, and epiphysis fractures; these can all be represented very well sonographically. The older forms of fracture appear in older age, e.g., intra-articular fractures; these can no longer be reliably diagnosed with ultrasound and must therefore be assessed radiologically.

Falls and crashes (e.g., running against the wall, balls) are given as the accident mechanism.

When doing a physical examination, the pain can usually be localized very well, so that carpal injuries can usually be excluded clinically. The main pain point is usually above the distal radius, isolated ulnar fractures are rare (<1% of cases). A swelling in the side comparison also indicates a bony injury. If there is no adequate trauma in children from the age of running or if there is anamnestic evidence of a systemic disease (e.g., osteogenesis imperfecta), an X-ray control is indicated, since these pathologies cannot be reliably visualized sonographically.

Furthermore, injuries of the hand and fingers as well as the forearm shaft and proximal forearm fractures must be clinically excluded.

8.4 Contraindications and Indications for X-ray Diagnostics

In the case of open injuries, the ultrasound examination is contraindicated in order not to cause any additional pain and to not apply any ultrasound gel to the wound.

If a vascular or nerve injury is suspected, sonography should not be carried out, since complex injuries are to be expected here and rapid further radiological diagnostics, including sectional imaging, must be carried out. The additional benefit of sonography is limited here, so we do not recommend using it in these cases.

If a clear surgical indication is already given during the clinical examination, sonography is superfluous. At the current point in time, we recommend preoperative X-ray diagnostics for planning the procedure for all planned operations so that one of the rare complex damage patterns (e.g., debris zones) is not overlooked. This also applies if the surgical indication is only made sonographically.

If the finding cannot be reliably assessed, the diagnosis can be verified by displaying different levels (see examination). If there is still no clarity, an X-ray examination is indicated. This is usually the case at the beginning of the application of fracture sonography and is rarely necessary for the experienced examiner. However, it is better to make your own diagnosis and to take an additional X-ray picture than to delay the process with repeated checks and to unsettle therapists and patients with unsafe diagnostics. Such an X-ray check also serves to confirm your own sonographic diagnosis and thus to gain certainty in the assessment of findings.

If no fracture is primarily diagnosed sonographically, an X-ray check should be carried out for 5 days if symptoms persist. A new sonography will show no result other than the primary examination and is therefore unnecessary. In such a case, the wrist should also be examined again so that no fracture is overlooked. If the pain is centered here, an MRI is indicated, since X-rays cannot adequately display carpal fractures in children.

X-ray diagnostics should also be carried out in the event of refractions, especially if there is no adequate trauma, in order to rule out pathological processes (cyst, osteomyelitis, foreign bodies, bone formation, or healing disorders). At the moment, there is insufficient experience with fracture sonography for refractures, so we recommend the historical gold standard here.

8.5 Examination

Diagnostics and therapy follow the Wrist SAFE algorithm.

After taking the medical history and the clinical examination, the sonographic examination follows. Due to the uncomplicated storage and the cooling ultrasound gel, this is on average less painful than the X-ray examination.

8.5.1 Positioning

The little patient sits on the examination couch, next to or on the lap of the parents. It is generally not necessary to darken the room. The affected wrist is stretched out when prompted, usually in a relieving pronation. No further positioning is necessary during the examination; the transducer is moved around the wrist.

8.5.2 Sections

Since the examination usually starts intuitively at the dorsal radius, it makes sense to first examine the radius in all three

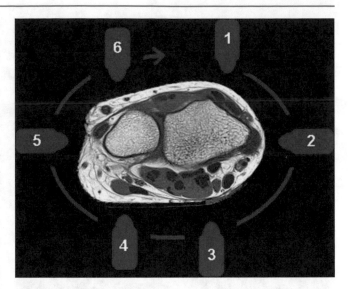

Fig. 8.2 Wrist examination planes. (©Ackermann and Eckert 2015; Courtesy of off label media)

planes (dorsal, radial, volar) and then the ulna in all three planes (volar, ulnar, dorsal). However, the procedure is left to the examiner according to individual preference (Figs. 8.2).

8.5.3 Setting

Finding the bones is never a problem, only the volar ulna is deep in the soft tissues, so that the beginner does not always succeed here. After showing the bone, which is shown as a bright, sharp line, the transducer is first aligned parallel to the longitudinal axis. This can be seen from the fact that the bone is shown across the entire width of the image section. Then the epiphyseal plate is shown. The correct setting has now been reached. The process is repeated in principle on all six levels, but experience has shown that this is very easy after the first setting.

8.5.4 Assessment

A fracture presents itself as a kink, bulge, offset, or fracture gap (Figs. 8.3, 8.4, 8.5, and 8.6). A special form is the edge break when abused (Fig. 8.7). A measurement of the axis deviation is based on the physiological course of the cortical and is at least as accurate as a radiological assessment. If the parallel setting is correct, an axis deviation can be underestimated, but not overestimated. Therefore, the greatest axis deviation can be set by swiveling and moving the transducer and this can be measured as true deformation (Fig. 8.8). It can therefore be assumed that these measurements are closer to the actual deviation than radiologically measured values, but there is no scientific evidence in larger series.

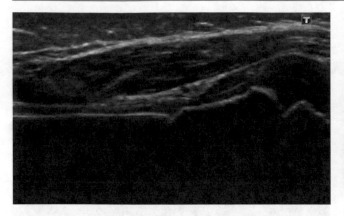

Fig. 8.3 Types of fractures: fracture gap. (©Ackermann and Eckert 2015; Courtesy of off label media)

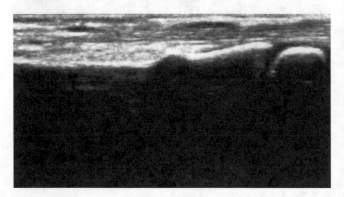

Fig. 8.4 Fracture shapes: bulge. (©Ackermann and Eckert 2015; Courtesy of off label media)

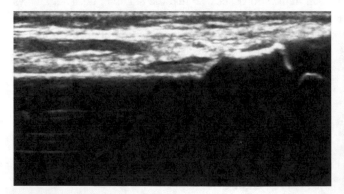

Fig. 8.5 Fracture shapes: offset. (©Ackermann and Eckert 2015; Courtesy of off label media)

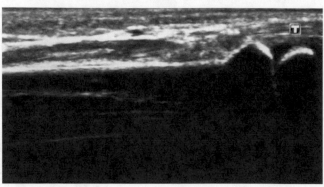

Fig. 8.6 Fracture shapes: kink. (©Ackermann and Eckert 2015; Courtesy of off label media)

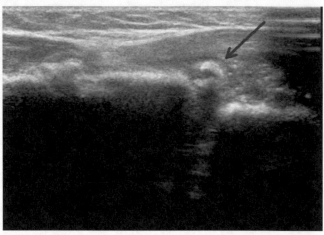

Fig. 8.7 Fracture shapes: edge breaking off with abuse. (©Ackermann and Eckert 2015; Courtesy of off label media)

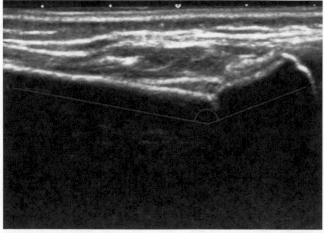

Fig. 8.8 Measurement of axis deviation. (©Ackermann and Eckert 2015; Courtesy of off label media)

It should be noted that all structures that are distant from the cortical bone are artifacts. Due to the large difference in impedance and the total reflection at the cortex, areas behind it cannot be assessed (Fig. 8.9).

If an undisplaced or little postponed epiphysiolysis is suspected, the healthy opposite side can also be examined. Here, the focus of the assessment is on the distance between the epiphyseal nucleus and the bone edge (Figs. 8.10 and 8.11); this is measured and compared in all three levels. An additional X-ray examination has no advantage here.

8.5.5 Diagnosis

The diagnosis is made purely sonographically and, if the axis deviation is not tolerable, followed by the reposition and, if necessary, stabilization under anesthesia. Before an operation, we currently recommend an X-ray examination on two

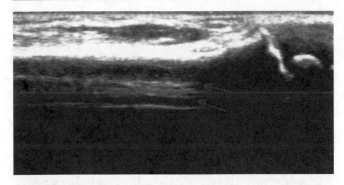

Fig. 8.9 Repetition artifacts. (©Ackermann and Eckert 2015; Courtesy of off label media)

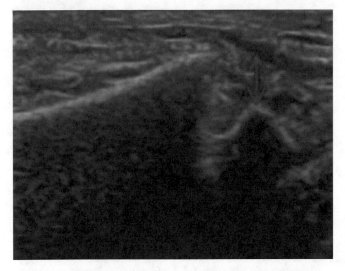

Fig. 8.10 Epiphysiolysis on the wrist. (©Ackermann and Eckert 2015; Courtesy of off label media)

levels, e.g., to reliably record any multifragmentary zones and special cases.

Radiological clarification is also carried out if other osseous pathologies such as an osteitis, cyst, or the like are suspected.

With all uncertainties in the diagnosis, the additional X-ray examination is permitted.

8.5.6 Therapy and Controls

The therapy is based on the generally known guidelines for distal forearm fracture in growing age. With conservative indications, the pain-adapted immobilization in the forearm plaster takes place in our own procedure, due to the mostly stable fractures even with complete forearm fractures only in exceptional cases with an upper arm cast. We only perform sonographic position checks if there is evidence of a dislocation clinically (inspectorally or due to increased pain), which is rarely the case. A sonographic consolidation check is also not mandatory if there is no clinical pressure pain.

If no fracture is diagnosed sonographically, the therapy is pain-adapted. If the discomfort is discrete, treatment is carried out functionally; if there is significant pain or a bony pressure pain (pressure pain of the bone if it is palpated from several directions), a cast is applied. All of these patients are checked on the fifth day after the accident. If there is still pressure pain over the radius or ulna or swelling at this point, an X-ray check is carried out in two planes; if the result is bland, the therapy is completed.

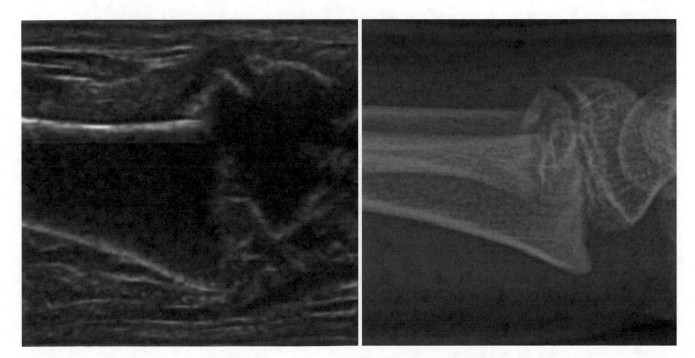

Fig. 8.11 Epiphysiolysis/Aitken I fracture in comparison. (©Ackermann and Eckert 2015; Courtesy of off label media)

8.6 Pitfalls and Red Flags

8.6.1 Ulna from Volar

It is sometimes difficult for the beginner to depict the ulna from volar because it is comparatively deep in the soft tissues. A representation of this level should not be left out. With increasing experience, the problem disappears on its own.

8.6.2 Undislocated Epiphysiolysis

The problem of displaying this injury is known from radiological imaging, which such a lesion cannot represent either. The procedure is analogous to that for radiological diagnostics. Since it is an undislocated injury, conservative therapy can be used. In most cases, an X-ray check is carried out after the Wrist SAFE on day 5 because pain persists; however, this shows an identical finding. If further therapy is carried out with pain-adapted immobilization, no problems are to be expected.

8.6.3 Carpal Injury

These cannot be reliably diagnosed or ruled out sonographically or radiologically. At the latest on the fifth day, a carpal injury is clinically distinguishable from an injury to the long forearm bones. If there is a suspicion of a relevant carpal injury, an MRI is the diagnostic of choice.

8.6.4 Proximal Forearm Injuries

These injuries are rare in childhood, but combination injuries should be considered. An additional proximal fracture or an Essex-Lopresti lesion, which may well have its maximum pain on the wrist, should be clinically excluded. If suspected, an X-ray check of the affected region is carried out.

8.6.5 Systemic Diseases

Broken bones or refractions without adequate trauma, previous operations with a septic component, signs of inflammation or pre-traumatic symptoms as well as a family history indicate a deeper or systemic disease and should be clarified radiologically. Sonography always shows only the bone surface and the pathologies that can be identified there.

8.6.6 Increasing Pain/Spontaneous

Expression of Pain

If the symptoms increase with adequate therapy or if the child spontaneously reports pain in the cast, precise clinical control is mandatory. Instability should be ruled out clinically by new imaging and a pressure point in the plaster.

Further Reading

False-Negative Results Are Balanced in X-ray and Sono

1. Eckert K, Ackermann O, Schweiger B, Radeloff E, Liedgens P. Sonographic diagnosis of metaphyseal forearm fractures in children: a safe and applicable alternative to standard X-rays. Pediatr Emerg Care. 2012;28:851–4.

First Major Comparative Examination of X-ray/Sonography

2. Ackermann O, Liedgens P, Eckert K, Chelangattucherry E, Husain B, Ruchholtz S. Sonographische Diagnostik von metaphysären Wulstbrüchen. Der Unfallchirurg. 2009;112:706–11.

Meta-analysis of Fracture Sonography on the Wrist

3. Douma-den Hamer D, Blanker MH, Edens MA, Buijteweg LN, Boomsma MF, van Helden SH, Mauritz GJ. Ultrasound for distal forearm fracture: a systematic review and diagnostic meta-analysis. PLoS One. 2016;11:e0155659. https://doi.org/10.1371/journal.pone.0155659.

Exam Time and Cost Analysis

4. Katzer C, Wasem J, Eckert K, Ackermann O, Buchberger B. Ultrasound in the diagnostics of metaphyseal forearm fractures in children—a systematic review and cost calculation. Pediatr Emerg Care. 2016;32:401–7.

Wrist SAFE

5. Eckert K, Ackermann O. Fraktursonographie im Kindesalter. CME Fortbildung Der Unfallchirurg. 2014;117:355–68.

Fracture Sonography on the Wrist Is Less Painful than the X-ray Examination

6. Ackermann O, Emmanouilidis I, Rülander C. Ist die Sonographie geeignet zur Primärdiagnostik kindlicher Vorderarmfrakturen? Deutsche Zeitschrift für Sportmedizin. 2009;60:355–8.

Subcapital Fracture of Fifth Metacarpal

Ole Ackermann

9.1 Synopsis

1.1 Rationale of application: Determination of the axis deviation in subcapital metacarpal 5 fractures.
1.2 Evidence level: V.
1.3 Indication: unclear surgical indication for subcapital metacarpal 5 fractures.
1.4 Contraindications: vascular/nerve damage.
1.5 Age of the patient: any age.
1.6 Examination: longitudinal section of the volar and dorsal view.
1.7 Indications for additional X-ray diagnostics: unclear findings.
1.8 Pitfalls: Rotational deviations can be underestimated.
1.9 Red flags: rotation deviation when the fist is closed, increasing pain.

9.2 Introduction

In the case of subcapital metcarpal 5 fracture (boxer fracture), the indication for surgery is based on the dislocation. Since the metacarpal bones completely overlap in the strictly lateral X-ray plane, the X-rays are usually taken in dorsopalmar and oblique planes, so that no assessment is made in two planes at 90° to each other and the extent of the dislocation can be underestimated. Due to the overlapping of the metacarpal bones, the strictly lateral image is not always meaningful and also requires exact positioning, which can be difficult for children.

9.3 Indication Including Patient Age

The indication for sonographic assessment is given in all cases with an unclear surgical indication. Due to the problems of X-ray imaging, the findings should be confirmed sonographically with every decision regarding conservative therapy.

9.4 Contraindications and Indications for X-ray Diagnostics

If there is a clinically existing rotational error, the finding can often also not be recorded correctly sonographically, so that further radiological diagnosis is indicated here.

9.5 Investigation

9.5.1 Positioning

The patient is sitting or lying down, special positioning is not necessary.

9.5.2 Levels

It is shown as a longitudinal section of strictly dorsal and strictly palmar, the latter being far more meaningful.

9.5.3 Setting

After the bone is found, the transducer is positioned so that the cortices are displayed across the entire width of the screen. A shaft portion of the metacarpal 5, the metacarpal head and the metacarpophalangeal joint should be recorded in the image.

O. Ackermann (✉)
Department of Orthopedic Surgery, Ruhr-University Bochum, Bochum, Germany

© Springer Nature Switzerland AG 2021
O. Ackermann (ed.), *Fracture Sonography*, https://doi.org/10.1007/978-3-030-63839-9_9

9.5.4 Assessment

The essential level for assessment is the volar representation. The axis deviation can usually be represented very well here. To measure the deviation, the epiphyseal plate can be used in children, in adults the gentle arch of the metacarpal 5 cortex is interpolated distally, thus determining the dislocation.

Rotational errors must be clinically ruled out (fist closure) and cannot be reliably assessed sonographically.

9.5.5 Diagnosis

The diagnosis is made on the volar level; the dorsal level serves to confirm the deviation and is not meaningful enough on its own.

9.5.6 Therapy and Controls

If conservative treatment or stabilization with antegrade intramedullary wires is used, the position checks can also be carried out sonographically. It should be kept in mind, that a dislocation of the wires is not clearly vivid in ultrasound examination.

9.6 Pitfalls and Red Flags

Rotational errors cannot be reliably assessed sonographically. If the bone is previously damaged, measuring the dislocation can be difficult or impossible.

A cast has to be removed for ultrasound examination.

9.6.1 Red Flags

The rotation should also be checked during the course. In the event of an unstable situation even after an operation (e.g., in the case of comminuted fractures), the position should be checked radiologically, since plaster removal is not feasible.

Injury to the PIP Joint of the Fingers: Fibrocartilago Palmaris

Thierry Kponton

10.1 Synopsis

1.1 Rationale of application: X-ray-free diagnosis and therapy of injuries to the palmar plate of the fingers.

1.2 Evidence level: V.

1.3 Contraindications: open injuries, Suspicion of vascular/nerve damage, luxation, instability, or clearly visible malposition.

1.4 Age of the patient: no age limit.

1.5 Examination: longitudinal view from palmar and dorsal.

1.6 Indications for additional X-ray diagnostics:
   - evidence of dislocation.
   - joint instability or dislocation.
   - uncertainty in the assessment.
   - large bony tearing fragments or evidence of further fractures.
   - scheduled operation.

1.7 Pitfalls:
   - open epiphyseal plate of the proximal middle phalanx.
   - shaft fractures.
   - impression fractures of the articular surface.
   - injuries to the ring bands or collateral bands.

1.8 Red flags:
   - severe pain/immobility without proof of fracture.
   - dislocation of the joint with instability, subluxation, or reluxation after reduction.
   - increasing complaints under therapy.

10.2 Introduction

Lesions of the PIP joints of the fingers are common injuries and are treated regularly in every traumatological practice and in the clinic. The main causes are impact trauma during ball games or a fall on the outstretched fingers [1]. Accordingly, the peak of injuries is in children of school and young adults. In most cases, hyperextension in the PIP joint of the affected finger is reported. Clinically there is typically a spindle-shaped thickening of the PIP joint with more or less hematoma and painful loss of movement. In the clinical examination, the maximum of pain is located at the PIP joint, so that shaft fractures of the phalanges can usually be excluded clinically (Fig. 10.1).

The slightly curved bone and the thin soft tissue make the joint easily accessible for sonographic imaging. Difficulties can arise with a high-grade extension deficit or with very small fingers in relation to the transducer.

The examination is painless and can be carried out quickly. For the experienced examiner, the sonographic examination takes about 1 min. A comparison with the non-injured finger next to the affected one can be carried out without repositioning and is generally recommended.

So far, the gold standard is X-rays in two planes. Our own observations indicate that the rate of false-negative results in ultrasound diagnostics and X-ray imaging are identical. Small fractures can be masked by the overlay of the bones on the X-ray image; sometimes small, undisplaced bony fragments of the Fibrocartilago palamaris are not shown on the

T. Kponton (✉)
Praxisklinik Orthopädie und Chirurgie München-West,
Munich, Germany
e-mail: dr.kponton@chirurgie-orthopaedie.de

© Springer Nature Switzerland AG 2021
O. Ackermann (ed.), *Fracture Sonography*, https://doi.org/10.1007/978-3-030-63839-9_10

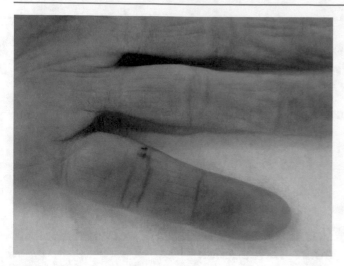

Fig. 10.1 Typical swelling and palmar hematoma when the PIP joint is injured

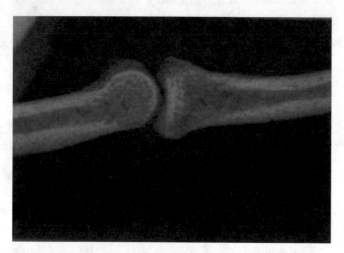

Fig. 10.2 Conventional X-ray finger PIP joint

ultrasound. However, since the vast majority of patients can be treated conservatively [2, 3], these missed findings do not seem to be of medical importance if they are treated based on clinical findings and the joint is correctly immobilized in a stretched position (Fig. 10.2).

10.3 Indication

Impact or twisting trauma of the fingers with pressure pain and swelling over the PIP joint are common. The extent of the injury can usually be assessed well on ultrasound. The sonographic diagnosis of fingers is an ideal screening method for both children and adults. Sonography is also very suitable for monitoring the treatment in order to diagnose a fragment dislocation of a primarily undisplaced fragment. Due to the large number of patients, a large number of X-ray examinations can be avoided, especially in the radiation-sensitive childhood. The indication for primary sonography of the PIP joint can thus be made widely.

10.4 Contraindications and Indications for X-ray Diagnosis

If a clear surgical indication is already given during the clinical examination, sonography is superfluous. In the case of open joint injuries, the ultrasound examination is contraindicated in order to avoid the contamination of the wound with ultrasound gel. In case of a manifest joint instability (sub- or reluxation) or persisting luxation, an X-ray examination p.a. and strictly laterally is carried out. Likewise for misaligned fingers with a maximum pain in the area of the phalanges or dorsally on the PIP joint. Such an X-ray control also serves to confirm your own sonographic diagnosis and thus gain certainty in the assessment of findings and will become less necessary with increasing experience.

If no fracture is primarily diagnosed sonographically, an X-ray check should be carried out after 5 days if symptoms persist despite adequate immobilization with extended PIP joint.

10.5 Examination

After taking the medical history and the clinical examination, the sonographic examination follows. Due to the uncomplicated positioning and the cooling ultrasound gel, this is usually less painful than the X-ray examination.

10.5.1 Positioning

The patient sits in a chair next to the examination table. It is generally not necessary to darken the room. The affected hand is placed in supination on the examination table, the fingers are stretched. In rare cases, if the affected finger cannot be stretched sufficiently due to pain, padding and hyperextension of the wrist can often improve the finger position.

10.5.2 Views

Typically, the transducer is placed palmar in the middle of the longitudinal axis on the stretched finger. In the event of a suspect bony finding in the area of the base of the middle phalanx, the finding can be assessed additionally by a parallel shift in ulnar and radial direction as well as rotating the transducer in the longitudinal axis by a few degrees. The examination is completed by a dorsal plane to rule out a rare edge fracture. However, the procedure is left to the examiner according to individual preference. If a phalanx fracture is suspected, two additional lateral levels from ulnar and radial direction are carried out (Figs. 10.3, 10.4, and 10.5).

10.5.3 Setting

Finding the joint never causes problems. After displaying the phalanges, which appear as a bright, sharp line, the transducer is first aligned parallel to the longitudinal axis. This can be seen from the fact that the cortex of the proximal and middle phalanx present across the entire width of the image section. Then the joint gap is centered in the center of the picture. The correct setting has now been reached. The process is repeated dorsally. In addition, the basic phalanx including the metacarpophalangeal joint and the middle phalanx with DIP joint can be assessed in case of appropriate symptoms (Figs. 10.6 and 10.7).

10.5.4 Assessment

The usually existing intracapsular hematoma offers a good contrast, so the distal basic phalanx, the joint space, the

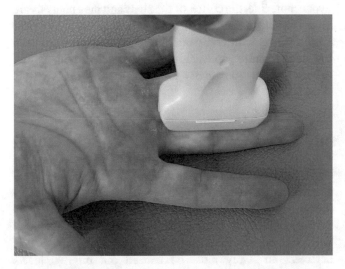

Fig. 10.3 Positioning

proximal central phalanx, and the fibrocartilago palmaris can be assessed well with the overlying flexor tendons (Fig. 10.8).

A small, or slightly displaced, bony tear of the fibrocartilago palmaris (types 1 and 2 according to Hintringer and Leixnering) cannot always be visualized by sonography. If the finding cannot be assessed with certainty, the diagnosis can be verified by displaying a different view and comparing it with the normal finding in an uninjured finger. More dislocated or larger fragments (types 3–6) can be easily recognized. They are not to be confused with the epiphyseal plate, which is located on the phalangeal base, i.e. on the PIP joint distal to the joint space. They can be seen in children up to around the age of 15 [4] (Figs. 10.9, 10.10, 10.11, 10.12, 10.13, 10.14).

10.5.5 Therapy and Controls

The aim of the treatment is a pain-free, freely movable, and stable PIP joint. The indication for surgery should be used with caution so as not to add an additional treatment trauma to the injury trauma [5].

It is essential that the joint is stretched to counteract fibrosis and shrinking of the palmar plate. In the case of significant hyperextensibility, a forearm finger splint or a dorsal PIP splint is recommended. Otherwise, the finger is taped to the next healthy finger or the joint immobilized by a finger splint. The duration of treatment is 2–4 weeks, depending on the findings. For larger fragments, a referral to a specialialist in hand surgery is advised to decide on the need for surgical intervention (Figs. 10.15 and 10.16).

A fragment that is not or only slightly displaced should initially be checked for dislocation as part of a tape or splint check, with sonography ideally carried out by the same examiner (check after approx. 4, 7, and 11 days). At this point, after the acute pain has decreased, the passive hyperextensibility of the joint should also be checked as a sign of

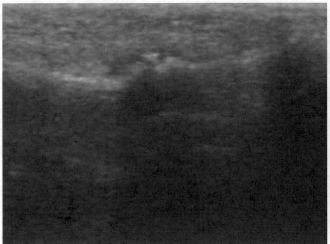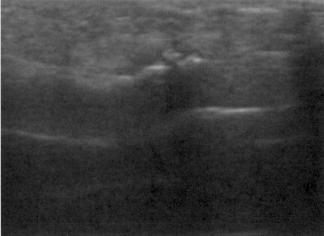

Figs. 10.4 and 10.5 Small bony tear of the fibrocartilago different imaging when tilting/rotating the transducer

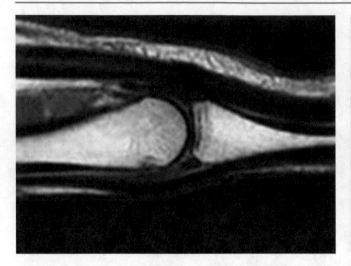

Fig. 10.6 MRI (with the kind permission of the Radiological Group Practice in Leipzig)

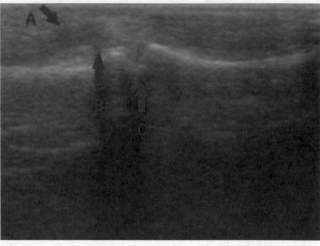

Fig. 10.8 PIP joint with intracapsular hematoma (A = flexor tendon, B = intracapsular hematoma, C = PIP joint)

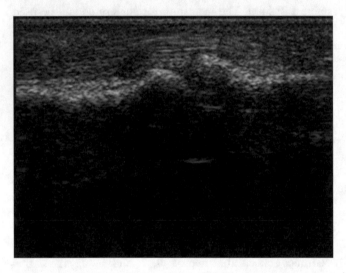

Fig. 10.7 Sonography finding of an uninjured PIP joint

instability, since this finding might require surgery, despite the lack of a bony lesion. I do not recommend the investigation in local anesthesia advocated by some authors [6].

10.6 Pitfalls and Red Flags

10.6.1 Open Epiphyseal Plate

The growth plates are detectable in children up to around the age of 15. They can be found at the phalangeal basis. Sonographically, it is always recognizable as a vertical,

hypoechoic line, the cortex of the shaft and the epiphysis are on one level. In the case of a fragment of the appropriate size, a tilting with corresponding step formation and/or a low-echo fracture gap can always be detected. With careful extension, the movement of the fragment is visible (Fig. 10.17).

10.6.2 Shaft Fractures

Shaft fractures can often be identified during the clinical examination. In addition to a malposition that is not always recognizable due to the swelling, the manipulation of the fractured diaphysis is quite painful. Even minor malpositions can be visualized sonographically. If a fracture is detected, an X-ray must be carried out on two levels (Fig. 10.18).

10.6.3 Injuries to the Ring Bands

In contrast to lesions of the fibrocartilago palmaris (impact trauma), ring ligament injuries in the area of the PIP joint are primarily caused by maximum tension with extended DIP and flexed PIP joint (climbing). The A2 ring band is most frequently affected, less often the A4 and A3. The typical "bow-stringing," i.e., the bow-string-like lifting of the flexor tendons, which otherwise run close to the bone, can be clearly recognized by sonography, which in the dynamic examination can be up to 10 mm (normal <2 mm) [7].

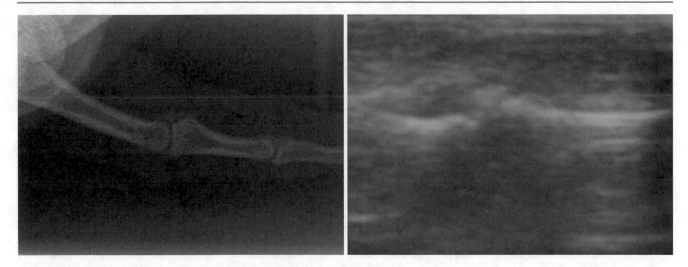

Figs. 10.9 and 10.10 Larger bony tear of the fibrocartilago at the PIP with little dislocation

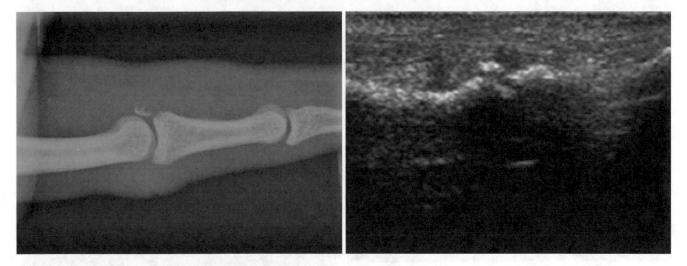

Figs. 10.11 and 10.12 Dislocated, shell-like bony tear of the fibrocartilago at the PIP

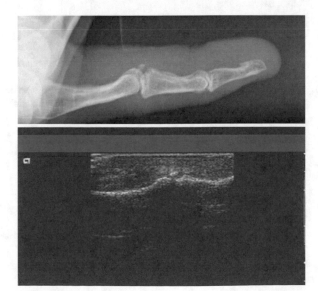

Figs. 10.13 and 10.14 Moderately dislocated tear of the fibrocartilago at the PIP

10.6.4 Severe or Increasing Pain

Due to hematoma of the articular capsule PIP lesions can be very painful and some patients show a gentle posture with completely eliminated movement. Especially in children, it might need some experience to differentiate between "not wanting to move" and "not being able to move."

If the symptoms increase with adequate therapy, clinical control is essential. If this has not already been done, a conventional X-ray of the finger should be arranged on two levels. If there is a radiological suspicion of a complex lesion with an impression of the articular surface, even a thin-layer CT or an MRI may be necessary for clarification and the patient should be referred to a specialist in hand surgery.

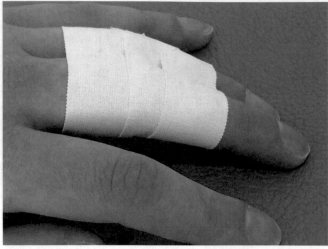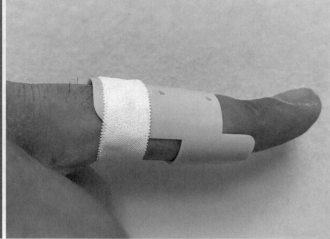

Figs. 10.15 and 10.16 Immobilization of the PIP joint in extension with tape and prefabricated finger splint

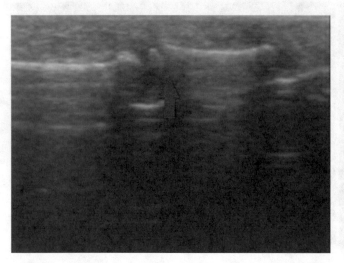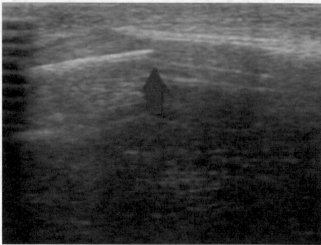

Fig. 10.17 Normal finding of a PIP joint with an open epiphyseal plate

Fig. 10.18 Fracture of the base phalanx from dorsal

References

1. Pillukat T, Mühldorfer-Fodor M, Schädel-Höpfner M, Windolf J, Prommersberger K-J. Verletzungen der Mittelgelenke. Unfallchirurg. 2014;117:315–26.
2. Hintringer W, Leixnering M. Knöcherne oder ligamentäre Verletzungen am Mittelgelenk und ihre Behandlung. Handchir Mikrochir Plast Chir. 1991;23:59–66.
3. Rudolf K-D. Operationsindikation bei Verletzungen der palmaren Platte des Mittelgelenkes. Orthopäde. 2008;37:1187–93.
4. Schuster W. Kinderradiologie 1, Bildgebende Diagnostik. Berlin: Springer; 1990.
5. Prommersberger K, Lanz U. Verletzungen des Fingermittelgelenkes. I. Frische Verletzungen. Akt Traumatol. 1999;29:246–53.
6. Schaller P, Geldmacher J, Landsleitner B, Aldebert D. Rupturen der palmaren Platte—konservative oder operative Therapie. Handchir Mikrochir Plast Chir. 1989;21:322–7.
7. Kluge S. Ultraschalldiagnostik der Hand. Berlin: Springer; 2015. p. S146–7.

Sternoclavicular Dislocation

11

Ole Ackermann

11.1 Synopsis

1.1 Rationale of application: initial diagnosis, detection/exclusion of dislocation, and instability.
1.2 Evidence level: V.
1.3 Indication: initial diagnosis if SC dislocation is suspected.
1.4 Contraindications: acute shortness of breath.
1.5 Age of the patient: any age.
1.6 Examination: cross-section over both SC joints; stability test by pressing the clavicle.
1.7 Indications for additional X-ray diagnostics: dorsal dislocation, uncertainty of the assessment.
1.8 Pitfalls: a side comparison is mandatory; clinically, it is often not possible to differentiate it from the sternum fracture, and the sternum should also be examined.
1.9 Red flags: shortness of breath, persistent pain, or persistent instability.

11.2 Introduction

Sternoclavicular dislocation is a rare injury and is usually triggered by an accident. The assessment is difficult or impossible in terms of native radiology because the superposition of the sternum and ribs usually does not allow a reliable diagnosis. Sonography is, therefore, the method of choice for confirming the clinical suspicion and for correctly indicating the diagnosis of a sectional image. If the situation is stable and/or there is a ventral dislocation of the clavicle, a CT scan may be dispensed; however, if an instability or dorsal dislocation occurs, the subsequent sectional imaging is mandatory.

11.3 Indication Including Patient Age

If there is a clinical suspicion of sternoclavicular dislocation, the indication for fracture sonography is given at any age. Since the clinical symptoms are similar to those of a sternal fracture and differentiation is not always possible, the indication for the examination of the sternum is given widely. This happens regularly in our own approach.

11.4 Contraindications and Indications for X-ray Diagnostics

In acute respiratory distress, CT diagnosis should be carried out without delay in order to rule out dorsal dislocation and pneumothorax.

If a dorsal dislocation is demonstrated, a sectional image is necessary to exclude mediastinal injuries; if instability is present, a CT scan should be performed to clarify the need for surgery.

Further radiological imaging should also be carried out if the sonographic findings are unclear.

11.5 Investigation

11.5.1 Positioning

The examination is carried out in the supine position with the linear transducer.

11.5.2 Levels

The examination takes place on an anteroposterior level.

O. Ackermann (✉)
Department of Orthopedic Surgery, Ruhr-University Bochum, Bochum, Germany

11.5.3 Setting

After the bone has been found, the transducer is positioned transversely to the sternal manubrium; If the transducer is wide, both SC joints can be displayed in this way, otherwise, both SC joints are examined one after another (Figs. 11.1, 11.2, and 11.3). Since the joints can appear differently in different patients, the side comparison is mandatory here.

If the sternum is then to be clarified, the setting is made in the longitudinal direction of the sternal body.

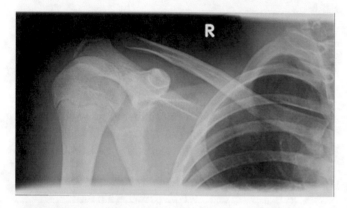

Fig. 11.1 X-ray examination of an SC dislocation on the right. (©Ackermann and Eckert 2015; Courtesy of off label media)

11.5.4 Assessment

Any side difference is suspect of an injury to the SC joint. To test the instability, the pressure is exerted on the clavicle with the transducer, and abnormal mobility is assessed in a side comparison (Fig. 11.4).

If a representation is not possible, the radiological diagnosis is carried out.

11.5.5 Diagnosis

The diagnosis of dislocation is made in a direct side comparison, as is instability.

11.5.6 Therapy and Controls

In the case of a dorsal dislocation, the further therapy decision is made after the CT diagnosis. If an operation is planned with ventral instability, a CT is also recommended here to assess the fragment situation for planning the operation. In the case of conservative therapy, the controls for callus formation and joint stability can be carried out sonographically, but no experience has been gained with surgical therapy.

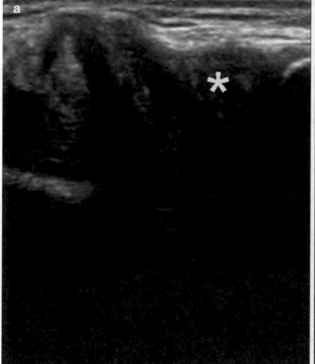
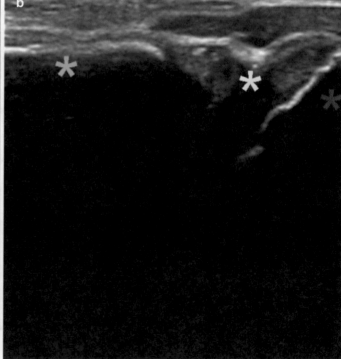

Fig. 11.2 Same patient as in Fig. 11.1. Side-comparative representation of the SC joints (**a** right, **b** left). Green marking: sternum; yellow marking: SC joint; red marking: clavicle on the left, which does not appear on the right. This leads to the suspicion of a dorsal dislocation of the clavicle. (©Ackermann and Eckert 2015; Courtesy of off label media)

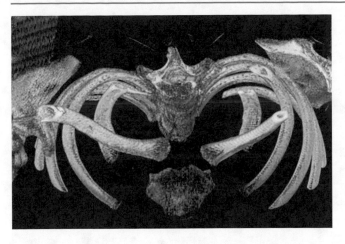

Fig. 11.3 Same patient as in Figs. 11.1 and 11.2. CT confirmation of the dorsal luxation of the right clavicle. (©Ackermann and Eckert 2015; Courtesy of off label media)

11.6 Pitfalls and Red Flags

A side comparison is always mandatory; If the SC joints cannot be visualized, a radiological examination is recommended.

A fracture of the manubrium or corpus sterni is usually not clinically distinguishable from an SC lesion, which is why an examination of the sternum is indicated. In order not to overlook a (very rare) combination lesion, the standard visualization of the sc-jont and the sternum makes sense for every examination.

As acute shortness of breath can have various, even acutely life-threatening causes (e.g., pneumothorax, mediastinal injury) that cannot be diagnosed reliably using sonography, sectional imaging should be initiated immediately.

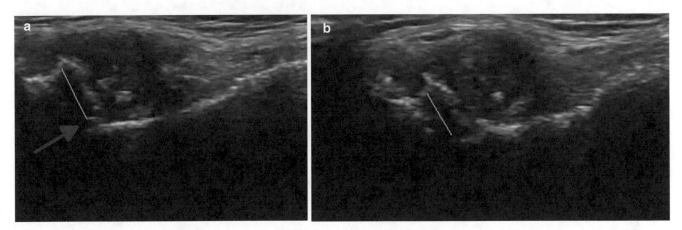

Fig. 11.4 (a) Stability check for ventral clavicular dislocation on the right, without pressure. Red arrow: SC joint; green marking: distance between the front edge of the clavicle and sternum. (©Ackermann and Eckert 2015; Courtesy of off label media). (b) Stability check with ventral clavicular dislocation on the right, with pressure. Green marking: reduced distance between the front edge of the clavicle and sternum. (©Ackermann and Eckert 2015; Courtesy of off label media)

Rib and Sternal Fractures

Christoph F. Dietrich

12.1 Synopsis

1.1 Rationale of use: diagnostics of rib and sternum fractures and accompanying injuries.
1.2 Evidence level: Ib.
1.3 Indications: suspect of rib or sternal fracture.
1.4 Contraindications: unstable patients.
1.5 Age of the patient: any age.
1.6 Examination: clinical limitation of ROI, targeted sonographic examination in longitudinal section; exclusion of accompanying injuries.
1.7 Indications for additional X-ray/CT diagnostics: high-grade dislocation, evidence of accompanying injuries.
1.8 Pitfalls: clinically overlooked rib fractures, pneumothorax, mediastinal injuries.
1.9 Red flags: shortness of breath, cardiac symptoms, hemodynamic instability, worsening of findings in the course.
1.10 Algorithm: not standardized.

12.2 Introduction

On the one hand, sonographic fracture diagnosis on the chest has established itself as a highly sensitive and precise method in some centers, but on the other hand, it is not yet used sufficiently frequently in everyday life [1, 2].

The value of chest sonography to assess the ribs and sternum has been underestimated by the assumption that the bone itself and the air content of the lungs are general obstacles to ultrasound. However, a large number of pathological changes in the chest wall, pleura, and lungs can be visualized sonographically, including fractures of the ribs and sternum and their complications. Due to the variability in sonographic planes, post-traumatic lesions can be visualized based on the pain symptoms and the necessary punctures and tissue removal can be carried out promptly [2–5].

The conventional X-ray diagnosis (chest X-ray examination) is particularly uncertain on the thorax and symptom-oriented, and therefore, targeted sonography at the pain point is particularly helpful. If the findings are unclear, computed tomography is the method of choice [2, 6].

The special value of chest ultrasound diagnostics lies in primary diagnostics as well as in differential diagnostics and progress monitoring, detection of complications, and the prompt intervention option (e.g., ultrasound-controlled biopsy). An adequate interpretation of the sonographic findings is always made in connection with the clinic and any radiological findings that may exist.

12.3 Indication Including Patient Age

The indication for sonography is determined by the injury mechanism, the severity of the trauma, the symptoms, and cooperation of the patient. Sonography is indicated for mild and moderate trauma, tolerable pain, and conscious and therefore, cooperative patients. Complications such as hematothorax, pneumothorax, and contusions can usually be safely delineated around the fracture if they are not overlaid by air or bone.

In general, sonography is superior to conventional X-ray diagnostics for mild and moderate trauma and can therefore generally be used as a primary diagnostic tool.

12.4 Contraindications and Indications

The severe trauma requires standard computed tomography diagnostics. CT is, therefore, indicated for severe trauma, severe pain, impaired consciousness, and noncooperative

C. F. Dietrich (✉)
Kliniken Hirslanden Beau Site, Salem und Permanence, Bern, Switzerland
e-mail: c.f.dietrich@googlemail.com, christophfrank.dietrich@hirslanden.ch

© Springer Nature Switzerland AG 2021
O. Ackermann (ed.), *Fracture Sonography*, https://doi.org/10.1007/978-3-030-63839-9_12

patients. In the case of severe trauma, complications deep in the thorax can occur and cannot be detected with sufficient certainty by sonography. In particular, the severity of a pneumothorax cannot be determined sonographically. CT is also indicated if there is a discrepancy between the severity of the complained symptoms and unclear sonographic findings.

The importance of conventional X-ray diagnostics is shaped by local customs and the quality of the examination technique. Conventional X-ray diagnostics lead to a large number of uncertain findings. It has been abandoned in a few centers, but is also standard diagnostics in many trauma-surgical processes. The cooperative patient is suitable for the sonographic examination, with an alcoholized or uncooperative patient conventional X-ray diagnosis is preferable. Clinical experience in the choice of diagnostics is crucial.

12.5 Examination

The chest wall and the parts of the lungs close to the chest wall are usually examined with higher-frequency transducers (5–18 MHz). When assessing the lungs via the subcostal and parasternal access route, 3.5–7 MHz transducers with a handy transducer contact surface are helpful for better depth penetration (convex or sector transducer with a narrow aperture).

The examination sequence follows the patient's pain information. The patient's position is determined by the symptoms and the clinical context; the region of interest should be easily accessible and the examination position should be as painless as possible for the patient.

By gentle compression with the transducer, minor fracture signs can be objectified on the one hand and the plasticity of accompanying changes (e.g., fluctuating internal echoes of fluid accumulations) can be assessed [3, 7].

12.5.1 Positioning

Depending on the suspected injury, the examination can be carried out on the lying, standing, or sitting patient in sonographic planes adapted to the findings.

The examination does not require any special preparation and can also be carried out in the intensive care unit for seriously ill patients.

In the case of ventral pain location, the examination is usually carried out in a supine position, but can also be carried out while sitting, or in individual cases, while standing. By raising the arm in the neck or to the shoulder of the opposite side, the intercostal spaces are spread and the scapula is rotated externally. This means that areas that are primarily covered by the scapula can also be examined [2–5].

12.5.2 Sonographic Views

In contrast to X-ray diagnostics, chest sonography is not assessed based on planes (e.g., transverse, coronary, or sagittal planes), but based on anatomy and topography. All pathological findings are shown in at least two planes.

12.5.3 Setting

The described pain allows targeted examination at the fracture site. The adjustment is made based on the bone structures in their longitudinal plane so that the cortex is shown over the entire width of the ultrasound image; further monitoring of the anatomical course is also possible. The patient's indication of pain is crucial for the correct detection of the fracture. Knowledge of anatomy and, for example, the epiphyseal plates is crucial for the correct assessment of the findings.

12.5.4 Assessment

Bone fragments can be safely visualized. In addition to the direct fracture signs with the discontinuity of the cortex with a step or gap formation, the accompanying findings, in particular, can also be reliably displayed. These include periosseous hematoma, pleural effusion, pneumothorax, and lung contusion foci.

In the case of very discreet fractures and undetectable discontinuity of the cortex without the formation of gaps and steps, the detection of a repetition artifact helps, which was also called "chimney phenomenon" in the literature. This reverberation artifact, which is associated with individual comet tails, arises at the interfaces of the fragments and reaches a variable depth. Undisplaced rib fractures can also be unmasked (with appropriate analgesia) using gentle pressure based on the pathological motility.

On the ribs as well as on the sternum, physiological findings at the cartilage-bone border should not be confused with a fracture; knowledge of anatomy and the clinical symptoms help here.

In patients with a suspected diagnosis of a rib fracture in the event of trauma, sonographically, significantly more rib fractures can be identified than with the chest X-ray [4].

12.5.5 Diagnosis

The pathological changes in the chest wall are characterized according to their position, size, shape, contour, morphology, and echo pattern, based on their compressibility and deformability as well as their relationship to the environment. Normally, sonographically identical symmetrical smooth interfaces are impressive. Due to the high acoustic impedance jumps, only the limitation of the bones and the

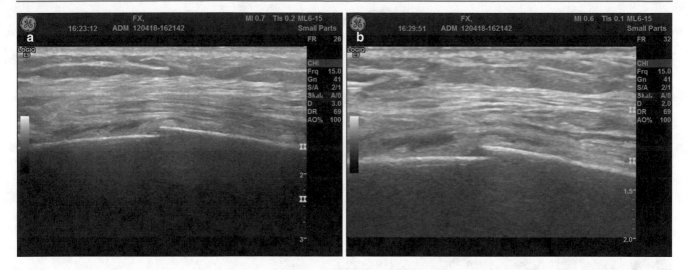

Fig. 12.1 The main criterion for a rib fracture is the representation of the fracture gap (**a**). The optimization of the penetration depth and focus are shown here (**b**)

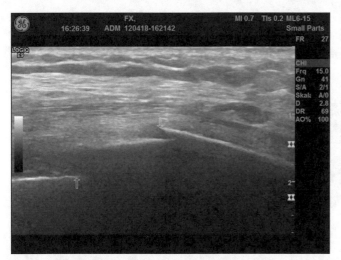

Fig. 12.2 The main criterion for a rib fracture is the representation of the fracture gap (upper arrow). Lung slippage is also evaluated (lower arrow) to correctly identify a pneumothorax

air-containing organs can be assessed. The description of the echo pattern and the morphology therefore often only refers to the pathological finding (e.g., fracture and its complication [2–5, 7, 8].

12.5.5.1 Rib Fracture

The rib fracture is searched for with the help of the patient's pain and is reliably identified based on the bone discontinuity. The rib fractures are examined parallel to the course of the bone. At the point of pain, the bone-oriented examination is performed by variable layers that are based on the discontinuity of the bone surface (Figs. 12.1, 12.2, 12.3, 12.4, and 12.5).

12.5.5.2 Sternum Fracture

The sternum fracture is targeted by the pain indication and reliably recognized based on the bone discontinuity. The

sonographic detection rate of the sternum fracture is higher than in the conventional X-ray image (Fig. 12.6).

12.5.5.3 Rib Contusion

The differentiation of a fracture compared to a simple rib contusion is possible due to the lack of fracture detection and may also have sociomedical consequences.

12.5.5.4 Lung Contusion

Foci of lung contusion (e.g., circumscribed bleeding) can be suspected sonographically.

12.5.5.5 Hematoma

The hematoma around a fracture is usually less echogenic than the surrounding area, but can also be isoechogenic, or more echogenic than the surrounding area during acute hemorrhage. Bone healing (callus formation) can be recognized by reactive and convex contour changes with acoustic shadows. After healing, there is a convex, differently delimited sound reflex zone on the newly formed cortex [3, 7].

12.5.5.6 Pneumothorax

The rapidly available sonography also enables targeted diagnostics if a pneumothorax is suspected. The pneumothorax can be detected sensitively, but the extent cannot be determined.

Air in the pleural space can be detected sonographically sensitively [2, 4, 9, 10]: the pleural reflex band is broadened by the air in the pleural space and the respiratory movement of the lungs and breathability of the pleura can only be demonstrated to a limited extent or not at all [2, 9, 10]. As a further criterion, the air-related subpleural reverberation echoes (repeat echoes) may be missing. The side comparison with the opposite side is important. It should be borne in mind that the extent of air expansion in the pleural space

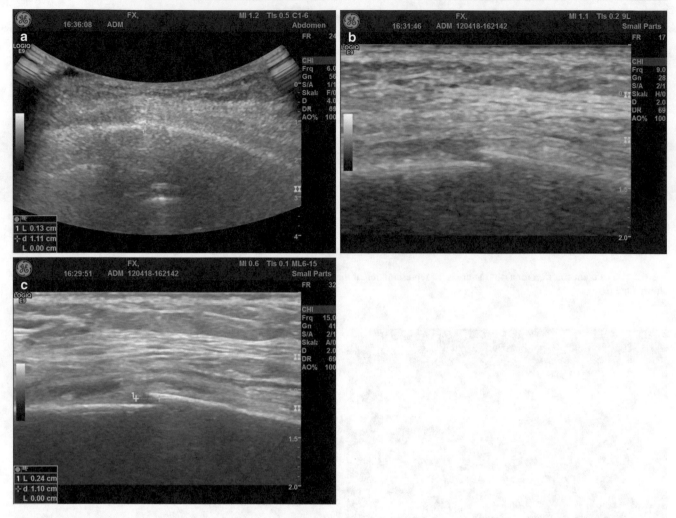

Fig. 12.3 Optimized device technology allows reliable diagnosis. The following image sequence shows (**a**) rib fracture with a curved array transducer (the fracture is in the area of the markers, hardly visible) with a higher frequency transducer (9 MHz), (**b**) an adequate high-frequency transducer (15 MHz), and (**c**) only the higher-frequency transducers allow the fracture to be displayed correctly with improved resolution

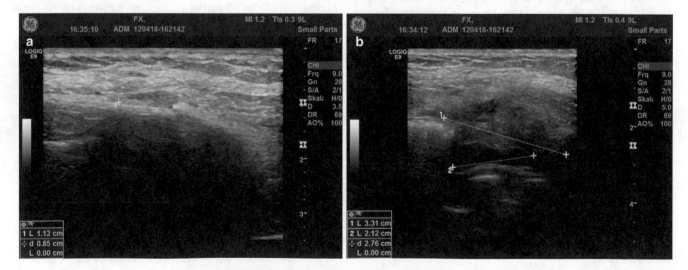

Fig. 12.4 (**a**) The main criterion for rib fractures is the representation of the fracture gap and the accompanying changes. (**b**) The accompanying hematoma and pleural effusion in the vicinity must be specifically sought and complete the sonographic image

Fig. 12.5 (**a**) Elastography enables the documentation of the relative tissue hardness to each other and (**b**) The contrast medium mode increases the sharpness of detail by displaying the harmonic frequencies

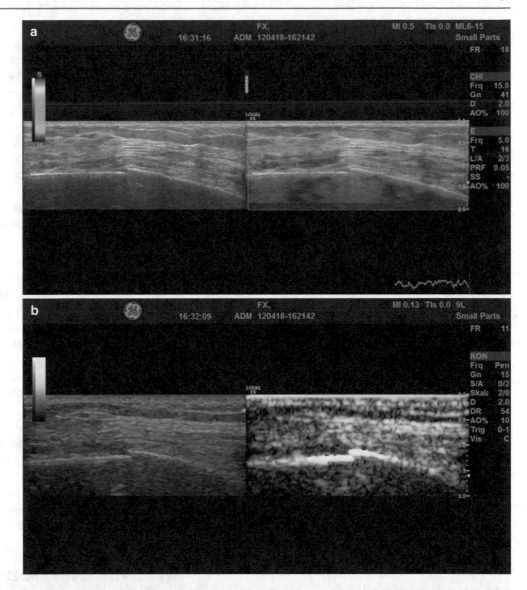

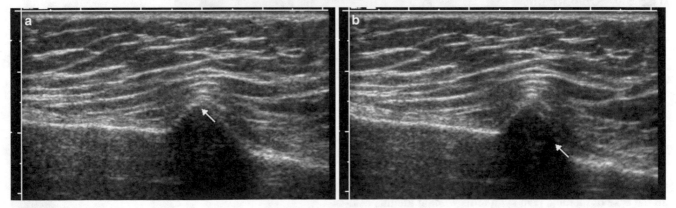

Fig. 12.6 Sternal fracture. The mobility of the fracture gap during respiration (inspiration (**a**) and expiration (**b**)) is shown and can be recognized by the change in angle

and lung collapse cannot be determined sonographically. A haematothorax, hematopericardium, and diaphragmatic ruptures can be reliably detected in the traumatized patient. Air inclusions can be recognized by the position-variable bright air reflections.

12.5.5.7 Pleural Effusion

Small pleural effusions are usually best detected in expiration in the posterior and lateral costodiaphragmatic recess in the seated patient. Smallest amounts (5–10 mL, e.g., small, breathable, circulated effusion quantities in pleuritis with color subdural blood flow that can be demonstrated by color Doppler sonography) can be punctured quickly and specifically under sonographic view. As a rule, a rough division of the pleural effusion into small, moderate, and extensive amounts of the effusion is sufficient, whereby the clinical findings (shortness of breath) and also the extent of secondary changes, for example, compression atelectases, are included in the assessment [3, 7].

The cause and composition of a pleural effusion cannot be reliably determined sonomorphologically. A reliable differentiation from exudate, bleeding or chylous fluid is speculative solely based on sonographic criteria and can only be achieved by puncture and additional examinations of the fluid obtained [3, 7]. Echogenic pleural effusions and septa are indications of bleeding.

12.5.5.8 Atelectasis

Depending on the amount of effusion, compression atelectases are found in pleural effusions. A secondary pneumonic infiltration of atelectasis changes its appearance (onset and volume increase). The reflex becomes convex, they appear less variable in shape, often rigid, and less echogenic [3, 7].

12.5.5.9 Diaphragm

The breath-synchronous diaphragm movements can be displayed in real time. Restricted diaphragm mobility is found in post-traumatic changes. A paradoxical mobility of the diaphragm with inspiratory upward movement can be found in phrenic paralysis. The sonographic and computed tomographic accuracy for the detection of pathological changes in the diaphragm are comparable. However, sonography is superior to computed tomography when assessing movement disorders of the diaphragm [3, 7, 11, 12].

12.5.5.10 Differential Diagnosis, Osteolysis

In the case of thoracic pain symptoms without trauma, osteolysis or inflammatory processes (osteomyelitis, osteochondritis) can also be detected. Osteolytic metastases can generally be represented as weakly echogenic (compared to the environment) convex and often sharply delineated circumscribed masses with atypical vascularization [3, 7]. Rib osteolysis is found particularly in small cell bronchial carci-

noma and breast carcinoma, but also in prostate carcinoma and other tumor entities.

The indication of the sonographically targeted puncture is obvious since the needle can be guided specifically into areas with blood supply and a targeted biopsy can be carried out according to the guidelines.

Bone infiltration in peripheral bronchial carcinoma (Pancoast tumor) is described elsewhere. The assessment of the lymph node stations is also important in the case of underlying tumor disease and suspected or proven osteolysis [13–19].

12.5.5.11 Use of Trauma Sonography in the Emergency Room

Targeted sonography of the chest, pleura, and lungs has established itself in the emergency room. In addition to the direct signs on the bones, connective tissue, pleura, and in consolidated lung areas, artifacts can also be defined. The artifacts are important for the diagnosis of pneumothorax (especially non-moving A-line artifact) and interstitial lung syndrome (B-line artifact) [10, 20, 21].

12.5.6 Therapy and Controls

Stress-free and noninvasive sonography is also of particular importance for the course assessment since it can be carried out without radiation and is readily available to the doctor treating the patient. Chest sonography also allows a course assessment of rib fractures. Bone healing disorders can be visualized by the detectable defects and movements of the fragments. Bone fractures on the ribs and sternum heal over weeks and months.

12.6 Pitfalls and Red Flags

Skin emphysema can make the sonographic assessment options of deep-lying thoracic structures difficult or impossible [3, 7, 22]. Disadvantages of sonography are also the limited views near the clavicle and, generally speaking, posterior parts of fractures. Adequate training must be ensured [1, 23–26]. Lung sonography is subject to limits due to the bony chest wall. Sound reflection and sound absorption result in pronounced sound shadow zones with limited assessability of lower-lying structures as well as artifact formation (e.g., multiple reflections, ring-down artifact, mirror artifacts).

12.6.1 Red Flags

The severe trauma, the impaired consciousness, the noncooperative patient, and a discrepancy in the severity of the clinical and sonographic findings are indications for clarification using CT. This applies in particular to progressive pain, confusing malpositions, and pathologic findings without adequate trauma.

References

1. Dietrich CF, Goudie A, Chiorean L, Cui XW, Gilja OH, Dong Y, Abramowicz JS, et al. Point of care ultrasound: a WFUMB position paper. Ultrasound Med Biol. 2017;43:49–58.
2. Dietrich CF, Mathis G, Cui XW, Ignee A, Hocke M, Hirche TO. Ultrasound of the pleurae and lungs. Ultrasound Med Biol. 2015;41:351–65.
3. Dietrich CF, Braden B, Wagner TOF. Thorax- und Lungensonografie. Dt Ärzteblatt. 2000;97:A103–10.
4. Bitschnau R, Gehmacher O, Kopf A, Scheier M, Mathis G [Ultrasound diagnosis of rib and sternum fractures]. Ultraschall Med. 1997;18:158–161.
5. Dietrich CF, Hirche TO, Schreiber D, Wagner TO. [Sonografie von pleura und lunge]. Ultraschall Med. 2003;24:303–311.
6. Lambert L, Ourednicek P, Meckova Z, Gavelli G, Straub J, Spicka I. Whole-body low-dose computed tomography in multiple myeloma staging: superior diagnostic performance in the detection of bone lesions, vertebral compression fractures, rib fractures and extraskeletal findings compared to radiography with similar radiation exposure. Oncol Lett. 2017;13:2490–4.
7. Dietrich CF, Braden B. Lunge und Pleura. In: Dietrich CF, editor. Ultraschall-Kurs. Köln: Deutscher Ärzteverlag; 2006. p. 293–303.
8. Dietrich CF. Lungen- und Thoraxsonografie. In: Meckler U, editor. Ultraschall des Abdomens. Köln: Deutscher Ärzteverlag; 1998. p. 202–11.
9. Dietrich CF, Mathis G, Blaivas M, Volpicelli G, Seibel A, Atkinson NS, Cui XW, et al. Lung artefacts and their use. Med Ultrason. 2016;18:488–99.
10. Dietrich CF, Mathis G, Blaivas M, Volpicelli G, Seibel A, Wastl D, Atkinson NS, et al. Lung B-line artefacts and their use. J Thorac Dis. 2016;8:1356–65.
11. Ahn HJ, Lee JW, Kim KD, You IS. Phrenic arterial injury presenting as delayed hemothorax complicating simple rib fracture. J Korean Med Sci. 2016;31:641–3.
12. Walz M, Muhr G. [Sonographic diagnosis in blunt thoracic trauma]. Unfallchirurg. 1990;93:359–363.
13. Trenker C, Gorg C, Jenssen C, Klein S, Neubauer A, Wagner U, Dietrich CF. [Ultrasound in oncology, current perspectives]. Z Gastroenterol. 2017;55:1021–1037.
14. Dietrich CF, Jenssen C, Herth FJ. Endobronchial ultrasound elastography. Endosc Ultrasound. 2016;5:233–8.
15. Dietrich CF, Annema JT, Clementsen P, Cui XW, Borst MM, Jenssen C. Ultrasound techniques in the evaluation of the mediastinum, part I: endoscopic ultrasound (EUS), endobronchial ultrasound (EBUS) and transcutaneous mediastinal ultrasound (TMUS), introduction into ultrasound techniques. J Thorac Dis. 2015;7:E311–25.
16. Jenssen C, Annema JT, Clementsen P, Cui XW, Borst MM, Dietrich CF. Ultrasound techniques in the evaluation of the mediastinum, part 2: mediastinal lymph node anatomy and diagnostic reach of ultrasound techniques, clinical work up of neoplastic and inflammatory mediastinal lymphadenopathy using ultrasound techniques and how to learn mediastinal endosonography. J Thorac Dis. 2015;7:E439–58.
17. Dietrich CF, Saftoiu A, Jenssen C. Real time elastography endoscopic ultrasound (RTE-EUS), a comprehensive review. Eur J Radiol. 2014;83:405–14.
18. Jenssen C, Annema JT, Zels K, Dietrich CF. Endosonographische Evaluierung von Lunge und Mediastinum. End Heu. 2014;27: 37–44.
19. Hirche TO, Wagner TO, Dietrich CF. [Mediastinal ultrasound: technique and possible applications]. Med Klin (Munich). 2002;97:472–479.
20. Wastl D, Borgmann T, Helwig K, Dietrich CF. [Rapid diagnostic in the emergency unit: bedside sonography]. Dtsch Med Wochenschr. 2016;141:317–321.
21. Wastl D, Helwig K, Dietrich CF. [Examination concepts and procedures in emergency ultrasonography]. Med Klin Intensivmed Notfmed. 2015;110:231–239; quiz 240–231.
22. Schute L. [Pneumothorax and subcutaneous emphysema following rib fracture]. Dtsch Med Wochenschr. 2007;132:698; author reply 698.
23. Dietrich CF, Rudd L, Saftiou A, Gilja OH. The EFSUMB website, a great source for ultrasound information and education. Med Ultrason. 2017;19:102–10.
24. Cantisani V, Dietrich CF, Badea R, Dudea S, Prosch H, Cerezo E, Nuernberg D, et al. EFSUMB statement on medical student education in ultrasound [long version]. Ultrasound Int Open. 2016;2:E2–7.
25. Cantisani V, Dietrich CF, Badea R, Dudea S, Prosch H, Cerezo E, Nuernberg D, et al. EFSUMB statement on medical student education in ultrasound [short version]. Ultraschall Med. 2016;37:100–2.
26. Christiansen JM, Gerke O, Karstoft J, Andersen PE. Poor interpretation of chest X-rays by junior doctors. Dan Med J. 2014;61:A4875.

Sonographic Diagnosis of Pneumothorax

13

Armin Seibel

13.1 Synopsis

1.1 Rationale of application: X-ray-free diagnosis of the pneumothorax.

1.2 Evidence level: IIa.

1.3 Indication: X-ray-free diagnosis of the pneumothorax, intervention control, and immediate result control.

1.4 Contraindications: none.

1.5 Age of the patient: no age restriction.

1.6 Examination: four sagittal craniocaudal sections per hemithorax.

1.7 Indications for additional X-ray diagnostics: skin emphysema in the examination area.

1.8 Pitfalls: reduced lung sliding, due to chronic pulmonary pathology or pulmonary protective ventilation, subcutaneous emphysema, use of software for image optimization (unwanted artifact suppression), use of high sound frequencies.

1.9 Red flags: one-sided or bilateral lack of lung sliding, hemodynamic and/or respiratory insufficiency, and missing lung point.

1.10 Algorithm: Fig. 13.1.

Fig. 13.1 Algorithm to clarify the sonographic question "Pneumothorax" for one thoracic examination position. Diagnostic reliability is increased by several applications in different chest regions. In case of clinically probable pneumothorax without evidence of a lung point, additional radiological imaging is indicated in hemodynamically stable patients. ©A. Seibel. All rights reserved

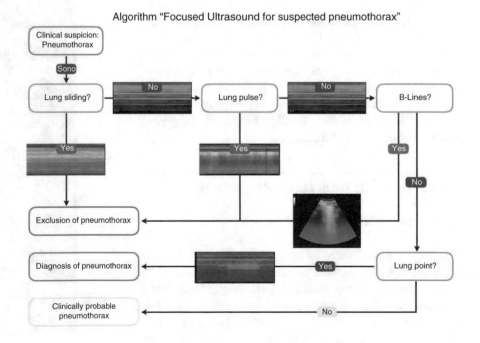

Algorithm "Focused Ultrasound for suspected pneumothorax"

A. Seibel (✉)
Department of Anesthesiology, Intensive Care and Emergency Medicine, Diakonie Klinikum Jung-Stilling, Siegen, Germany

© Springer Nature Switzerland AG 2021
O. Ackermann (ed.), *Fracture Sonography*, https://doi.org/10.1007/978-3-030-63839-9_13

13.2 Introduction

The term pneumothorax describes the condition of a patho-logical, extrapulmonary air accumulation in the thorax and represents a disease with considerable variability in terms of genesis, age distribution, and severity. A pneumothorax can be regarded as a so-called primary spontaneous pneumothorax, as well as iatrogenic, in patients previously regarded as healthy with lungs occur after thoracic or thoraco-vascular interven-tion or as a result of chest trauma. The incidence of spontane-ous pneumothorax is given in the literature as 22/100,000 inhabitants, which leads to approximately 10,000 hospitaliza-tions per year [1]. Men are affected by a factor of 3 more often than women. There is currently no reliable statistical informa-tion for pneumothorax, which is considered to be genetically independent.

Sonographic imaging has been well evaluated as a reli-able method of pneumothorax diagnostics and is comparable to CT in terms of diagnostic reliability [2, 3]. Although the method was published by Lichtenstein as early as 2000 [4] and since then has not undergone any relevant changes in terms of implementation and technical requirements, it is still mentioned in textbooks and guidelines as a new alterna-tive that should be reserved for those who have practiced sonography. This is mainly due to the fact that a thorough knowledge of the typical artifacts of lung ultrasound and their interpretation in the clinical context are necessary for the reliable sonographic diagnosis of a pneumothorax. Therefore, in addition to the pneumothorax diagnostic algo-rithm, the lung ultrasound artifacts lung sliding, lung pulse, B-lines, and the lung point are explained in their physical basis and significance. Basically, lung sliding, lung pulse, and B-lines can only be displayed if the ultrasound waves reach the surface of the lungs, which reliably excludes a pneumothorax, while the visualization of the lung point ensures the diagnosis of a pneumothorax.

13.3 Artifacts from Lung Ultrasound

13.3.1 Lung Sliding

The lungs are surrounded by the visceral pleura (pleura pul-monalis) and the parietal pleura (pleura costalis), which directly lines the parenchyma and the inner chest wall. There is a thin film of liquid between these two structures, which ensures low-friction sliding against each other as part of the ventilation-related expansion of the lungs. Since the ultra-sound in the medically usable frequency range is reflected completely due to the extremely large difference in imped-ance at the interface between tissue and air, the air-filled lung itself cannot be examined with ultrasound. The two pleural

sheets are clearly visible, however, since the total reflection of the ultrasound waves only occurs subpleurally in the alve-olar air. Although most ultrasound devices cannot display them as isolated anatomical structures due to their limited image resolution, the combination of the pleural sheets lying next to each other with the subpleural airogenic reflection surface leads to an easily representable hyperechogenic line that runs horizontally in the sonogram, the pleural line (Fig. 13.2). With breathing the movement of the visceral pleura, sonographically amplified by the air reflection sur-face, leads to a clearly visible flicker-like movement artifact of this hyperechogenic pleural line in the ultrasound image, the so called lung sliding. The visual strength of the lung sliding depends on the ventilation-related volume expansion of the lungs. For pragmatic image documentation, lung slid-ing in M-mode can be represented as a so-called seashore sign (Fig. 13.3). In this representation, the restless ("sandy") pattern below the pleural line corresponds to the movement artifact of lung sliding.

The depiction of lung sliding precludes the pneumothorax at the examined point since the air in the pleural space would inevitably prevent the visceral pleura from being depicted, and thus no lung sliding can occur in the sonogram in pneumothorax.

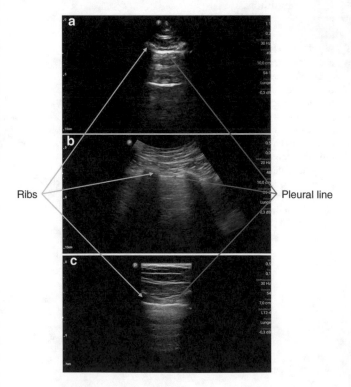

Fig. 13.2 Representation of the pleural line with a sector probe (**a**), a convex probe (**b**), and a linear probe (**c**). The pleura can be seen imme-diately below the ribs regardless of the ultrasound probe or sound-wave frequency used. ©A. Seibel. All rights reserved

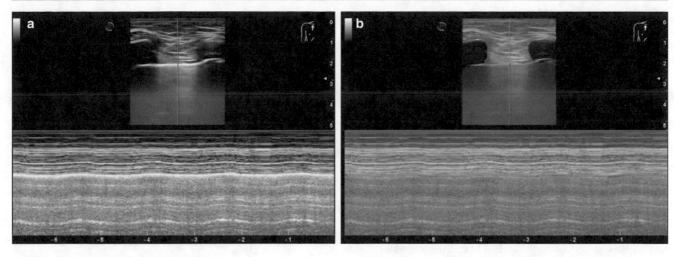

Fig. 13.3 "Seashore Sign" as documentation of the normal finding of lung sliding in M-mode. (**a**) In the color-coded illustration (**b**), the stratification of subcutaneous tissue (green; "Sky"), intercostal muscles (yellow; "Sea"), and the movement artifact of lung sliding (orange; "Beach") corresponding to the definition of the seashore sign is below the pleural line (highlighted in red). ©A. Seibel. All rights reserved

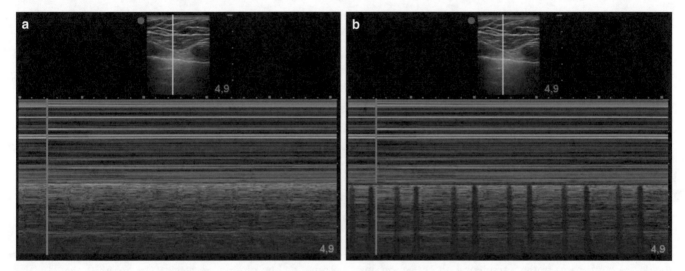

Fig. 13.4 Lung pulse in M-mode. (**a**) The vertical pulse-synchronous movement artifacts are limited by the pleural line (**b**, red line). When the M-mode sonogram is running at high speed and the heart rate is normal, the artifact lines can be assigned to the corresponding heart actions (atrium = light blue, chamber = dark blue). ©A. Seibel. All rights reserved

13.3.2 Lung Pulse

Pulse-synchronous movement of the pleural line that occurs independently of lung sliding is referred to as the lung pulse. The mechanical transmission of both myocardial contractions and the pulse wave in the arteries near the pleura down to the visceral pleura triggers a brief displacement of the pleural sheets against each other, which is expressed in the ultrasound image as a lung pulse.

If the sound conditions are good, the lung pulse can already be seen in the normal B-scan. To optimize diagnostic reliability and for documentation, however, it is advisable to display the lung pulse either in M-mode or through amplitude-coded color Doppler ("Power Doppler"). In M-mode, it

can be recognized as a pulse-synchronous vertical "fault line" line that extends from the lower edge of the picture to the pleural line (Fig. 13.4). When using the color Doppler, a pulse-synchronous flare of the Doppler signal, which is essentially limited to the pleural line and the subpleural area, can be represented in the moving image (Fig. 13.5).

The lung pulse thus also serves to exclude a pneumothorax.

13.3.3 B Lines

Owing to the minimal amount of alveolar fluid or edematous interlobar septa, subpleural punctual acoustic interfaces between fluid and alveolar air can arise, which can produce narrow echo rich artifacts. These artifacts, referred to as

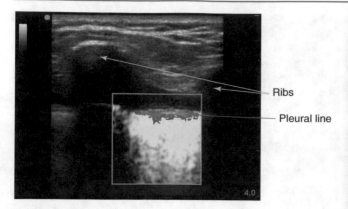

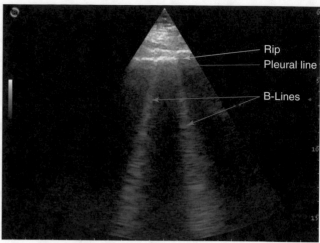

Fig. 13.5 Lung pulse in the amplitude-coded color Doppler (power Doppler). The still picture shows that the Doppler only detects the movement artifact below the pleural line. In such cases, the synchronicity with the pulse frequency can be seen in the moving image in contrast to the significantly slower movement frequency of the breath-synchronous lung sliding. ©A. Seibel. All rights reserved

Fig. 13.6 Thoracic examination with a sector probe. Two B-lines draw vertically from the pleural line to the end of the ultrasound image. In the moving image, these B lines follow the lung sliding. ©A. Seibel. All rights reserved

B-lines, range from the punctiform subpleural sound interface to the end of the sonogram in a laser-like manner and move synchronously with lung sliding (Fig. 13.6). The exact physical basis of the B lines has not yet been clarified. It is assumed that these reverberations arise as a high-frequency pendulum reflection between the interfaces involved.

The B lines only develop subpleurally and are therefore not visible when there is air in the pleural space. They also serve to exclude a pneumothorax.

13.3.4 Lung Point

In order to be able to detect pneumothorax sonographically, a special artifact, the so-called lung point, is required. This is the dorsal border area of the intrapleural air collection moving with breathing.

The lung point can only be visualized if the visceral pleura has not yet been completely detached from the inner thoracic wall by the air in the pleural space and is characterized in that both lung sliding and standing pleural line can be seen in the sonogram. In supine position, lung sliding moves a few millimeters from dorsal to ventral with each inspiration. The lung point is a specific lung ultrasond artifact that can only be found if a pneumothorax is present. An exception are extensive pneumothoraces, which have led to a complete circular separation of the pleural sheets. Since lung sliding can no longer occur in such situations, no lung point will be found either.

The lung point can also be documented pragmatically as an image in M-Mode. If the M-Mode marker is in an optimized position, the inspiratory movement pattern of the lung sliding (Seashore Sign) can be recognized as well as pure horizontal lines on expiration in the image as an expression of missing lung sliding (stratosphere sign) (Fig. 13.7).

13.4 Indication

Nowadays, there are many substantive and structural reasons for the use of sonography as the imaging method of the first choice in the suspected diagnosis of pneumothorax.

In comparison to conventional chest X-ray diagnostics, an advantage in terms of diagnostic certainty for lung ultrasound was demonstrated in several studies [5–7]. Lung ultrasound can also be performed at the bedside at any time and does not pose any high technical challenges for the device technology. This means that basically every available ultrasound device with sector, linear, or convex probe can be used for pneumothorax diagnostics since no special probe technology is necessary to reliably display the artifacts.

The indication for sonographic pneumothorax diagnosis should be very broad, because, on one hand, the pneumothorax may present a life-threatening illness, which should be diagnosed as soon as possible, on the other hand, this simple and ubiquitously available imaging is applicable without risk for the patient and at any age. In primary care for seriously injured patients, the E-FAST examination protocol (E-FAST = Extended Focused Assessment with Sonography in Trauma), which has been expanded to include pneumothorax diagnostics, has largely replaced the standardized FAST algorithm.

In traumatology, every form of chest trauma also requires focused lung ultrasound with the question of "pneumothorax". Even in situations in which the bony thorax appears to be undamaged, this suspected diagnosis remains until proof of exclusion since especially ribs in children or adolescents have greater flexural flexibility compared to older age, and therefore, lung parenchyma injuries can also occur without rib frac-

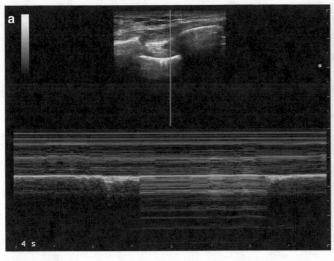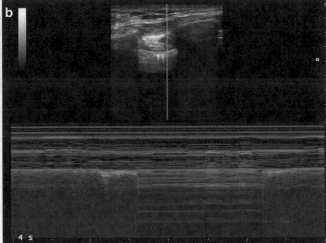

Fig. 13.7 (**a**) Lung point in M-mode. Here, the ultrasound probe is placed exactly at the boundary of the intrapleural air, which can be shifted by ventilation, so that lung sliding is still visible during inspiration, but no lung sliding is visible during expiration. (**b**) In M-mode the movement artifact of lung sliding ("Seashore Sign," orange) abruptly stops below the pleural line (red) and is replaced by the horizontal stripes of the "Stratosphere Signs" (green) as a correlate of an unmoving pleura. ©A. Seibel. All rights reserved

tures. In this context, it is noteworthy that the exclusion of a pneumothorax is one of the great strengths of sonography since only a few milliliters of air in the pleural space are sufficient to abolish the distinctive lung sliding. The simple detection of this lung sliding alone already allows the unequivocal exclusion of pneumothorax at the examined area.

However, blunt chest trauma also causes fractures of the bony thorax far more frequently, which in this context represents the most common injuries being more than 70%. Dislocated rib fractures are particularly worth mentioning as risk factors for parenchymal injuries with subsequent pneumothorax.

Further indications for sonographic pneumothorax diagnosis arise post-interventionally after performing thoracic procedures such as effusion drainage or vascular punctures for the placement of central venous catheters or venous ports. The risk of iatrogenic pleural injuries can be significantly reduced by the consistent use of sonographic puncture control, but it cannot be completely eliminated so that even in these cases, post-interventional focused lung ultrasound with the aim of excluding an iatrogenically generated pneumothorax should be carried out.

13.5 Contraindications and Indications for X-ray Diagnosis

Contraindications to performing focused lung ultrasound when pneumothorax is suspected does not exist, since sonography per se is not subject to any contraindications and especially in this emergency medical question, sonographic imaging should be the method of choice due to its high availability and diagnostic significance.

The sonographic answer to the question "pneumothorax" can, however, be restricted or even impossible under certain circumstances. Pronounced subcutaneous emphysema in the area of the chest wall can hinder sonography to such an extent that even the structures of the bony thorax can no longer be visualized. Unfortunately, especially in the case of highly acute pneumothoraces with a tension character, extensive skin emphysema often develops. In such situations, the examiner can try to push the subcutaneous air away for a few seconds with constant probe pressure, thus clearing the way for the ultrasound waves to the pleura. However, since the success of such a probe compression maneuver cannot always be achieved with certainty, there is an urgent indication for alternative radiological imaging.

In principle, for lung ultrasound as well as for any other sonographic question, there is an imperative to choose a second, alternative imaging method to optimize the diagnostic reliability if the findings are unclear. In lung ultrasound, uncertainties generally arise from the ambiguity of the necessary artifacts, which can be due to the clinical situation and errors in the device settings (see Sect. 13.7).

13.6 Examination

13.6.1 Positioning

The patient's position in the ultrasound diagnostics for pneumothorax doesn't matter. As a rule, affected patients with spontaneous breathing still preserved are in a seated or semi-seated position, while ventilated patients are usually in a

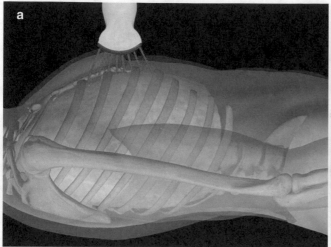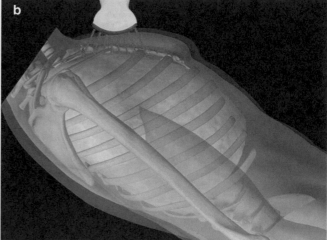

Fig. 13.8 (**a**) First thoracic standard examination point in supine position and suspected pneumothorax. (**b**) First thoracic standard examination point in semi-recumbent position and suspected pneumothorax. It should be noted here that the highest possible thoracic location point for

the detection of a pneumothorax in flat supine position lies much further caudal than when the upper body is in an upright position. ©A. Seibel. All rights reserved

supine position or with the upper body raised by 30°. However, sonographical examination of the lungs from dorsal and dorsolateral is also practicable in controlled ventilated intensive care patients who are in prone position because of the particular severity of their pulmonary disease.

Under the mechanistic assumption that if a pneumothorax is present, air will always collect in the pleural space at the highest point [8], the examination should, therefore, also begin at the top thoracic location point in relation to the patient's current body position (Fig. 13.8a, b).

Experience has shown, however, that when the patient is in a strictly seated position, the examination findings are often uncertain. The reason for this is that, on the one hand, there is less parenchyma expansion in the area of the cranial apex of the lung, and therefore, the important artifact of lung sliding is poorly developed, and on the other hand, free air is distributed both ventrally and dorsally to the apex of the lung, and the pneumothorax appears less pronounced as a result.

13.6.2 Probe Alignment and Regions of Examination

It is generally advisable to always start lung ultrasound in a sagittal plain and craniocaudal probe alignment (Fig. 13.9a). This sagittal standard plain enables reliable identification of the pleura, which is shown as a hyperchogenic line immediately below the two crosscut ribs (Fig. 13.9b). The main focus of this view is on demonstrating lung sliding. For the assessment of each lung ultrasound position, the immediately following examination at the mirror image position on the other side of the thorax is of great importance since differ-

ence of lung sliding in the direct side comparison can already give the first indication of a pneumothorax (Fig. 13.10a, b).

For a sufficiently precise focused examination, each hemithorax is divided into four regions (two ventrally, two laterally). For this subdivision, the intermammillary line serves as a horizontal subdivision line and the anterior axillary line serves as a vertical subdivision line (Fig. 13.11) [2]. In highly acute clinical situations, the examination can be reduced to two locations per hemithorax (positions 1 and 4 in Fig. 13.11) [9].

An intercostal alignment of the ultrasound probe is only of secondary importance in the context of the "pneumothorax" question since no diagnostic added value can be generated from this probe position in relation to the pneumothorax, whereas the lack of depth orientation due to the invisibility of the ribs in the intercostal window can lead to uncertainty in the assessment of the findings.

13.6.3 Setting

The ideal penetration depth is 7–10 cm regardless of the transducer selection. The pleural line is usually reached at a depth of 2–4 cm in the sonogram. For reliable detection of the artifacts B-lines or lung pulse, it is helpful to position the pleural line in the middle of the upper part of the sonogram (Fig. 13.9b).

Since the correct interpretation of the findings in lung ultrasound essentially depends on the reliable and clear presentation of the typical artifacts, it is advisable to switch off any image improvement to suppress artifacts on the ultrasound device (Compound Imagine, Tissue Harmonic Imagine) and to select sound frequencies below 10 MHz for the examination.

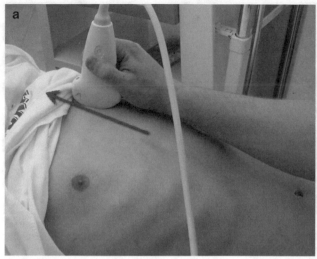

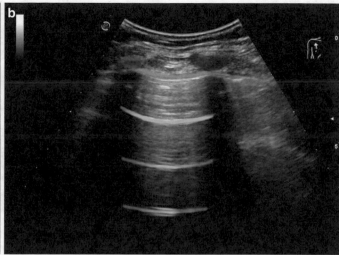

Fig. 13.9 (**a**) Cranio-caudal adjustment of the probe at the sagittal standard examination position. (**b**) Sonogram with correct adjustment of the probe. Two ribs are shown in cross section (blue), the left one marks the cranial, the right the caudal area. The pleural line (red) passes off directly under the ribs. The A-lines marked green in the sonogram are repeated echoes of the pleural line and have no diagnostic added value in pneumothorax diagnostics. ©A. Seibel. All rights reserved

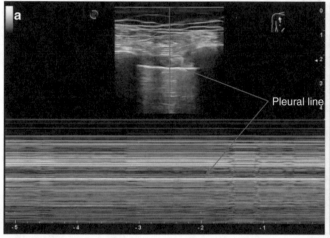

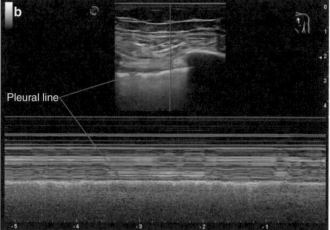

Fig. 13.10 Direct side comparison between the right and left side of the chest at a mirror-image examination position (here third ICR medio-clavicular). (**a**) The time course of this M-mode sonogram documents the horizontal line above and below the pleural line, which means that no echo reflexes from moving structures and thus no lung sliding was recorded (stratosphere sign). (**b**) This ultrasound image documents clear lung sliding on the left side of the chest using the "Seashore Sign." Although this side comparison does not yet prove pneumothorax, it allows urgent suspicion due to the lack of lung sliding on the right side and the considerable discrepancy to the left side. ©A. Seibel. All rights reserved

Even if in principle any common ultrasound probe (sector, convex, or linear probe) can be used, the peculiarities of the different probes must be taken into account. Experience has shown that lung sliding with the low-frequency sector probe often is less clear, whereas B-lines can best be represented with this probe. The high-frequency linear probe, on the other hand, shows lung sliding particularly clearly, but the high sound frequency leads to an underrepresentation of the B-lines and usually offers a less overview of deep structures than the other two probes. Since the sonographic question of pneumothorax occurs in most cases in connection with trauma, but almost always as an emergency medical question, it is usually clarified in the context of the standardized E-FAST examination procedure using the convex probe.

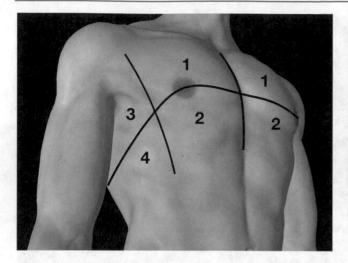

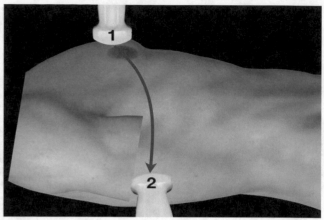

Fig. 13.11 Subdivision of the thoracic regions for the "pneumothorax" examination. Region 1 usually contains the highest chest point on a patient in supine position. If lung sliding can already be detected in this region using ultrasound, a clinically relevant pneumothorax on the examined side is excluded. Region 4 also allows a view of the dorsolateral thoracic area and thus early detection of intrathoracic free fluid. ©A. Seibel. All rights reserved

Fig. 13.12 Probe maneuvers for ventrally undetectable lung sliding and suspected pneumothorax. After documenting the missing lung sliding at the ventral examination position (1), the transducer is immediately moved as far dorsolaterally as the patient's position allows (2). If no lung sonographic artifact can be detected here either, an examination of the area between the two points makes no sense and would mean unnecessary investment of time. ©A. Seibel. All rights reserved

13.6.4 Assessment

As already described earlier, the detection of one of the three typical lung ultrasound artifacts lung sliding, B-lines, or lung pulse is sufficient to exclude a pneumothorax at the examination position. In a clinical situation where pneumothorax is suspected, the examiner should first focus on assessing lung sliding and only look for the other two artifacts when in doubt. In the case of lung sliding that is not clearly recognizable, the focus is initially on the representation of the lung pulse since only a heartbeat and the absence of air in the pleural space are necessary to detect it.

13.6.5 Diagnosis

If in a clinically compromised patient (dyspnea, hemodynamic instability), neither lung sliding, nor lung pulse or B-lines can be detected on one or both sides of the chest, the differential diagnosis "pneumothorax" becomes increasingly probable and can be confirmed if the lung point described in Sect. 3.5 is present (Fig. 13.1). As a goal-oriented examination strategy, it is advisable to reposition the transducer to the dorsolateral position as far as the patient's position allows (Fig. 13.12) after recognizing the fundamentally pathological situation based on the lack of lung sliding at the ventral position. If one of the artifacts can be shown here, at least a total collapse of the lungs on the examined side is excluded and you can now step back ventrally with the transducer to find

the lung point and thus prove the pneumothorax. Radiological control imaging is no longer indicated in this case.

If, however, no lung artifacts are still detectable at this posterior dorsolateral thoracic point, extensive pneumothorax must be assumed in connection with the patient's clinical symptoms and treated immediately with increasing hemodynamic and/or respiratory instability without waiting for further imaging.

In clinically (still) stable patients, additional radiological imaging should be performed to confirm the diagnosis in such situations.

13.6.6 Therapy and Controls

The typical target-oriented primary therapy for a pneumothorax is the sonographically controlled relief puncture and insertion of a small lumen drainage catheter (<14 CH) [10]. Adequate drainage of the ventral and ventro-apical intrapleural air in the patient in supine position can be done via two thoracic access routes:

1. Monaldi position: in the second intercostal space (ICR) in the medioclavicular line, and
2. In a modified Buelau position: in the fourth ICR in the anterior axillary line (the classic Buelau position in the posterior axillary line is used for transcutaneous drain of intrapleural hematomas or serous pleural effusions).

Continuous suction treatment via the inserted drain is particularly indicated for large amounts of intrapleural air that occur within minutes after an event, because with such progress, considerable lung parenchymal injuries resulting in leakages persisting over days must be assumed. After the thoracic drain has been successfully positioned, the lungs can expand again. This therapeutic success can be confirmed sonographically immediately after the intervention, even if lung sliding can be demonstrated again in the ventral thoracic sections.

However, not every pneumothorax requires therapy. In particular, small pleural leaks that have arisen spontaneously, as part of a thoracic trauma without accompanying rib fractures or post-interventionally iatrogenic, can also close again without therapy. In such cases, the intrapleural amounts of air are absorbed within a few days without the need for drain treatment. Such a development can also be reliably monitored on the bedside using ultrasound.

13.7 Pitfalls and Red Flags

As already described, a targeted interpretation of lung ultrasound findings can often only be achieved with the help of a reliable representation of the typical lung artifacts. However, a certain representation of artifacts can be compromised due to technical requirements, the peculiarities of acute medical situations, or examiner-dependent circumstances.

Since the lung sliding and lung pulse are movement artifacts of the lungs, no additional movement by the patient himself, a restless examiner's hand, or manipulations on the patient may be added during the examination. When using the transducer, it is also important to ensure that the direction of the soundwaves are aligned perpendicular to the surface of the lungs in order to achieve the sharpest possible representation of the pleural line.

In intensive care patients who are ventilated with lung protective ventilation pressures, there is only a slight tissue shift due to the low tidal volumes, which leads to a considerable reduction in lung sliding. Patients with pronounced emphysema also offer reduced lung sliding.

Pronounced pleural effusions can simulate an ultrasound finding similar to pneumothorax when using a linear probe since on the one hand no typical lung sliding sliding can be detected due to the intrapleural effusion liquid, but on the other hand, due to the limited penetration depth of the linear probe the effusion-related distance to the lungs cannot be overcome and the lung floating in the effusion is not shown.

The extent of a pneumothorax can only be assessed in ultrasound in terms of its extent over the surface, but not in depth. In the focused assessment of a pneumothorax that is not yet in need of intervention by closely monitoring the lung point, it is essential to ensure that the patient's body position is not changed. This aspect is becoming increasingly important due to the steadily growing spread of emergency ultrasound in the preclinical use since this increase in diagnostic certainty means that the initial diagnosis of a pneumothorax that may still be very discreet and therefore not (yet) in need of intervention can be made significantly earlier after an accident and sonography in the emergency room is the first control examination. If care is taken in the course of time between these two examinations to ensure that the patient's position is not changed significantly, a dorsal shift of the lung point in the emergency room can be regarded as a progression compared to the preclinical findings, which has a considerable advantage in the targeted emergency treatment.

References

1. Schnell J, Koryllos A, Lopez-Pastorini A, et al. Spontanpneumothorax. Dtsch Arztebl Int. 2017;114(44):739–44.
2. Volpicelli G, Elbarbary M, Blaivas M, et al. International evidence-based recommendations for point-of-care lung ultrasound. Intensive Care Med. 2012;38(4):577–91.
3. Xirouchaki N, Magkanas E, Vaporidi K, et al. Lung ultrasound in critical ill patients: comparison with bedside chest radiography. Intensive Care Med. 2011;37:1488–93.
4. Lichtenstein D, Meziere G, Biderman P, et al. The "lung point": an ultrasound sign specific to pneumothorax. Intensive Care Med. 2000;26:1434–40.
5. Hwang TS, Yoon YM, Jung DI, et al. Usefulness of transthoracic lung ultrasound for the diagnosis of mild pneumothorax. J Vet Sci. 2018;19(5):660–6.
6. Lichtenstein D, Goldstein I, Mourgeon E, et al. Comparative diagnostic performances of auscultation, chest radiography and lung ultrasonography in acute respiratory distress syndrome. Anesthesiology. 2004;100(1):9–15.
7. Rocco M, Carbone I, Morelli A, et al. Diagnostic accuracy of bedside ultrasonography in the ICU: feasibility of detecting pulmonary effusion and lung contusion in patients on respiratory support after severe blunt thoracic trauma. Acta Anaesthesiol Scand. 2008;52(6):776–84.
8. Mennicke M, Gulati K, Olivia I, et al. Anatomical distribution of traumatic pneumothoraces on chest computed tomography: implications for ultrasound screening in the ED. Am J Emerg Med. 2012;30(7):1025–31.
9. Lichtenstein D. Lung ultrasound in acute respiratory failure an introduction to the BLUE-protocol. Minerva Anestesiol. 2009;75(5):313–7.
10. AWMF, S3-Leitlinie "Diagnostik und Therapie von Spontanpneumothorax und postinterventionellem Pneumothorax". 2018). https://pneumologie.de/fileadmin/user_upload/010-0071_S3_Spontanpneumothorax-postinterventioneller-Pneumothorax-Diagnostik-Therapie_2018-03.pdf.

Distal Femoral Fracture

14

Ole Ackermann

14.1 Synopsis

1.1 Rationale of application: diagnosis and control of distal femoral torus fractures in childhood.
1.2 Evidence level: IV.
1.3 Indication: suspect of undisplaced distal femoral fracture in childhood.
1.4 Contraindications: vascular/nerve damage, visible axis deviation, polytrauma.
1.5 Age of the patient: up to 12 years.
1.6 Examination: longitudinal section in four planes (ventral, medial, dorsal, and lateral).
1.7 Indications for additional X-ray diagnostics: unclear findings, previous injuries, and suspect of abuse.
1.8 Pitfalls: femoral shaft fissures must not be overlooked.
1.9 Red flags: increasing pain, persistent stress insufficiency.

14.2 Introduction

Distal femoral torus fractures are benign fractures in childhood and can usually be treated conservatively. Since the fractures heal with a high correction potential and can be visualized sonographically, a sonographic diagnosis and control is possible.

14.3 Indication Including Patient Age

The indication for sonographic assessment is possible in children up to the age of 10 and in slim patients up to the age of 12. If the symptoms can be clinically narrowed to the distal femur after adequate trauma, an ultrasound-based treatment can be carried out first.

14.4 Contraindications and Indications for X-ray Diagnostics

If there are visible axis deviations, and therefore, the likely surgical indication, X-ray diagnosis is mandatory, and fracture sonography does not bring any advantage here.

In the case of bland sonographic findings and clinically unclear pain localization, an X-ray check should be carried out to exclude a fissure of the femoral shaft.

14.5 Investigation

14.5.1 Positioning

Since the femur is examined from all four directions, the patient is placed on his back with the knee bent at 90°.

14.5.2 Levels

It is shown as a longitudinal section in four planes from ventral, medial, dorsal, and lateral.

14.5.3 Setting

After the bone is found, the transducer is positioned so that the cortices are displayed across the entire width of the

O. Ackermann (✉)
Department of Orthopedic Surgery, Ruhr-University Bochum,
Bochum, Germany

screen. The epiphyseal plate and a small part of the knee should be recorded in the picture.

14.5.4 Assessment

The fracture is a cortical bulge and can usually be visualized on at least three levels. If there is a suspicion of a relevant axis deviation, the curved femoral cortex is interpolated distally or the epiphyseal plate is used for the measurement. Since this is not always possible, especially in the case of fractures close to the epiphyses, the dislocation should be measured radiologically in the event of uncertainty and therapeutic relevance.

14.5.5 Diagnosis

The diagnosis is made using classic sonographic fracture signs. If the course is uncomplicated, an X-ray diagnosis is not mandatory (Fig. 14.1a–d).

14.5.6 Therapy and Controls

If the treatment is conservative, the dislocations checks can also be carried out sonographically.

14.6 Pitfalls and Red Flags

With bland ultrasound findings and significant pain, a femoral shaft fracture must be clinically excluded; if this is not possible, an X-ray diagnosis should be carried out.

A splint hast to be removed for ultrasound control.

14.6.1 Red Flags

Persistent or increasing pain and persistent stress insufficiency give reasons for further radiological diagnosis in the case of bland sonographic findings.

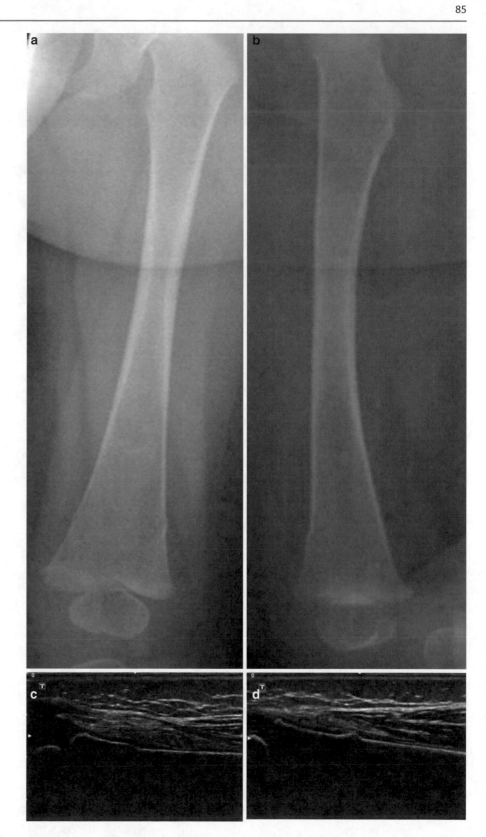

Fig. 14.1 Undislocated femoral bead fracture in radiological (**a**, **b**) and sonographic (**c**, **d**) imaging. (©Ole Ackermann 2020. All rights reserved)

Proximal Tibial Fracture

15

Ole Ackermann

15.1 Synopsis

1.1 Rationale for use: additional diagnostics in the event of clinical suspicion of a fracture and radiologically unclear findings.

1.2 Evidence level: V.

1.3 Indication: suspect of proximal tibia fracture in children up to the age of 12.

1.4 Contraindications: open fractures, vascular/nerve damage, clinically, or radiologically clear findings.

1.5 Age of the patient: for example, 0–12 years.

1.6 Examination: longitudinal section in four planes: tibia from ventral, ventromedial, dorsomedial, and dorsal.

1.7 Indications for additional X-ray diagnostics: always X-ray the fracture.

1.8 Pitfalls: progressive valgus deviation (Kadi fracture), pathological fracture, tumor.

1.9 Red flags: persistent pain, clinical signs of inflammation.

15.2 Introduction

The proximal tibia fracture in children can be treated conservatively in many cases. Torus fractures are often only discreet in the X-ray image. This is because the tibia is configured triangular and in the X-ray image, if there is no fracture gap, only the edges are shown, but the cortex surfaces are not (Figs. 15.1, 15.2, and 15.3). Therefore, in the case of torus fractures, only the outer extensions of the torus formation are shown, while the main finding is hidden behind the bone mass due to the overlay. There is usually a minimal bulge in the AP picture, while the side picture is completely unremarkable.

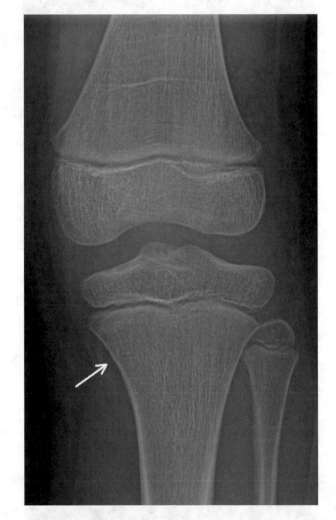

Fig. 15.1 X-ray tibial head a.p. X-ray of a 7-year-old girl with proximal tibial pain. Discrete bead medial in the a.p.picture. (©Ackermannn and Eckert 2015; Courtesy of "off label media")

Here, fracture sonography can quickly provide a reliable diagnosis and make the bulge clearly visible (Figs. 15.4, 15.5, and 15.6).

Since there are no randomized studies on this indication, the accompanying X-ray diagnosis is still mandatory.

O. Ackermann (✉)
Department of Orthopedic Surgery, Ruhr-University Bochum, Bochum, Germany

© Springer Nature Switzerland AG 2021
O. Ackermann (ed.), *Fracture Sonography*, https://doi.org/10.1007/978-3-030-63839-9_15

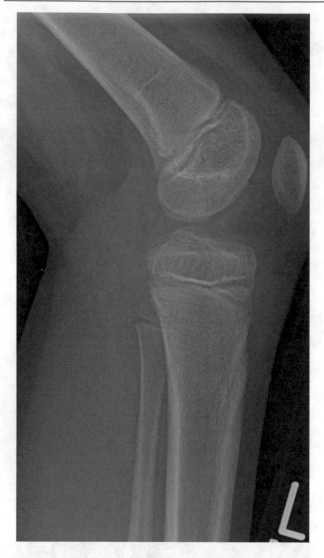

Fig. 15.2 X-ray of tibia head laterally. (©Ackermannn and Eckert 2015; Courtesy of "off label media")

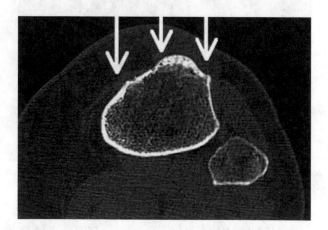

Fig. 15.3 Transverse CT in the case of a tibia head fracture; arrows: ray path in the a.p.-X-ray image (image tibia proximal cross-section). (©Ackermannn and Eckert 2015; Courtesy of "off label media")

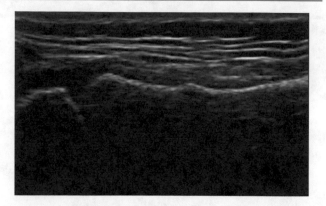

Fig. 15.4 Same patient as Figs. 15.1 and 15.2: ultrasound from ventro-lateral. (©Ackermannn and Eckert 2015; Courtesy of "off label media")

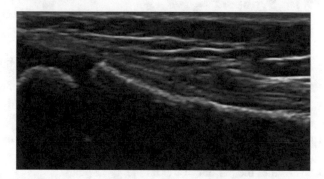

Fig. 15.5 Same patient as Figs. 15.1 and 15.2: ultrasound from ventro-medial. (©Ackermannn and Eckert 2015; Courtesy of "off label media")

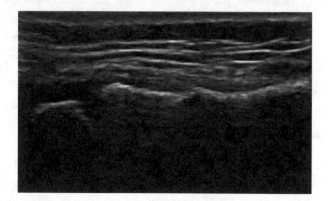

Fig. 15.6 Same patient as Figs. 15.1 and 15.2: ultrasound from dorsal. (©Ackermannn and Eckert 2015; Courtesy of "off label media")

However, it is to be expected that ultrasound can also be used for exclusion diagnosis at this point in the future and will also be used as sole imaging in the case of torus fractures. With gaping fracture gaps, long exposure for axis determination is always advisable.

15.3 Indication Including Patient Age

Accident mechanisms can cause falls, impact dreams, but also jumps from low altitude or trampoline jumps. The pain can usually be localized well, and there is usually an inability to walk. It is not uncommon for the patient to come to the examination after 1–2 days.

While bead fractures of the tibia head can be shown much better with ultrasound means in contrast to x-rays, there has been no experience to date of torn ligaments of the cruciate ligaments or hamstrings, tuberosity injuries, or epiphyseal joint lesions. For this reason, X-rays and ultrasound should always be done simultaneously if these lesions are suspected.

In the future, it is to be expected that the sole sonographic diagnosis will be sufficient for the benign torus fractures.

15.4 Contraindications and Indications for X-ray Diagnostics

Fracture sonography is limited to acute injuries. Since malignancies can also occur here, radiological control is always necessary for the event of long-lasting complaints or clinical signs of inflammation.

Even with gaping fracture gaps, the radiological axis check is mandatory in order to reliably detect a valgus malposition.

15.5 Examination

15.5.1 Positioning

Sitting or lying down, the entire knee must be free and accessible.

15.5.2 Levels

Ventral, ventromedial, dorsomedial, and dorsal; the lateral projection may not be adequately assessed by the overlying fibula.

15.5.3 Setting

Finding the bone is not a problem. After showing the bone, which is shown as a bright, sharp line, the transducer is first aligned parallel to the longitudinal axis. This can be seen from the fact that the bone is shown across the entire width of the image section. Then the epiphyseal plate is shown. The correct setting has now been reached.

15.5.4 Assessment

The torus is clearly evident in the first shot and can be followed around the circumference. A fracture hematoma can sometimes be visualized, but this is far from always the case.

15.5.5 Diagnosis

The diagnosis is currently being made in conjunction with the X-ray image. Radiological imaging is mandatoy in any case of doubt, especially if the findings are unclear.

15.5.6 Therapy and Controls

The treatment of torus fractures is conservative and unproblematic. Imaging controls are only necessary for clinical anomalies, otherwise, pain-adapted weight-bearing is allowed.

If the fracture gap is visible, radiological checks are mandatory so that a progressive valgus deviation is not overlooked.

15.6 Pitfalls and Red Flags

Owing to the combination of radiological and sonographic imaging, the examination is very safe and ultrasound-related complications are not to be feared.

15.6.1 Red Flags

Increasing pain, clinical axis deviations, atraumatic, or prolonged pain are reasons for further examinations. Inflammatory and neoplastic causes in particular must then be excluded.

A gaping fracture gap is always a reason for radiologic control since an axis deviation must then be excluded; no axis deviation is tolerable for this fracture.

Outer Ligament Tear at the Upper Ankle and Syndesmotic Tear at the Upper Ankle: "Lateral Collateral Ligament and Lateral Chain"

16

Norbert Hien

16.1 Synopsis

1.1 Rationale of application: X-ray-free diagnosis and therapy of fractures and capsular ligament injuries/instabilities in the area of the outer ankle and the lateral foot.

Differentiation from the most common accompanying injuries: peroneal tendons, inner ankle, delta ligament, and tibialis anterior and posterior tendon.

1.2 Evidence level: Ib for violations of the lig. fibulotalare anterius (FTA), tibiofibulare anterius (VS), and deltoideum (LD); IIa for the lig. fibulocalcaneare (FC) and calcaneocuboideum (CC). For violations of the lig. fibulotalare posterius (FTP), of the lig. tibiofibulare posterius (DS) and the osseous accompanying injuries in the area of the "lateral chain" can be assumed from an evidence level IIb to IV. So far, meta-analyzes of several randomized, controlled studies are missing, not least because of the still inconsistent examination techniques.

1.3 Indication: X-ray-free diagnosis and therapy control after sprains of the ankle and lateral foot if suspected capsular ligament injuries/instabilities or fractures of the ankle or hind and metatarsus.

1.4 Contraindications: open fractures with large or infection-prone skin and soft tissue damage.

1.5 Age of the patient: no age limit.

1.6 Examination:

	Structure	Section plane/ probe position	Examination technique	Question
1	Fibula	Longitudinal semi-circular	Dorsal, lateral, ventral	Fracture
2	MT5	Longitudinal semi-circular	Dorsal, lateral, ventral	Fracture
3	FTA	Transverse fibula to neck of the talus	Neutral stress anterior talus-drawer	Lesion signs instability >2 mm
4	AS	Transverse tibia-fibula	Neutral stress extension + external rotation	Lesion signs instability >1 mm
5	FC	Longitudinal along the ligament fibula to tub. innomin. calcanei	Neutral stress varus	Lesion signs instability >4 mm
6	CC	Longitudinal semi-circular calcaneus to cuboid	Lateral + dorsal stress add/sup	Lesion signs joint gapping
7	FTP	Transverse along the ligament	Neutral	Lesion signs
8	PS	Transverse tibia to fibula	Neutral	Lesion signs
9	MM/LD	Longitudinal medial malleus along lig. deltoideum	Neutral semi-circular 3 parts of the ligament	Fracture lesion signs

MT5 metatarsale 5, *FTA lig.* fibulotalare anterius, *AS lig.* tibiofibulare anterius (anterior syndesmosis), *FC lig.* fibulocalcaneae, *CC lig.* calcaneocuboideum, *FTP lig.* fibulotalare posterius (posterior syndesmosis), *MM* malleus medialis tibiae, *LD lig.* deltoideum

Structure / section plane / examination technique / question:

1. Fibula / longitudinal, semicircular / dorsal, lateral, and ventral / fracture.
2. MT5 / longitudinal, semicircular / dorsal, lateral, and ventral / fracture.
3. FTA / transverse, fibula to neck of talus / neutral, stress anterior talus drawer / lesion signs, instability >2 mm.

N. Hien (✉)
Praxis für Orthopädie und Unfallchirurgie, Munich, Germany

4. AS / transverse, tibia to fibula / neutral, stress extension + external rotation / injury signs, instability >1 mm.

5. FC / longitudinal along the ligament, fibula tip to tub. innom. calcan / neutral, stress varus / lesion signs, instability >4 mm.

6. CC / longitudinal semicircular, calcaneus to cuboid / lateral + dorsal, stress add/supp / lesion signs, joint gapping.

7. FTP / transversal along the ligament / neutral / lesion signs.

8. PS / transverse tibia to fibula / neutral / lesion signs.

9. MM/LD / longitudinal MM + along the lig. deltoideum / neutral, semicircular, 3 parts of the ligament / fracture, signs of lesions.

1.7 Indications for additional X-ray diagnostics:

– Dislocated fracture of the fibula or tibia with suspected surgical indication.

– Planned surgery.

– To exclude intraosseous or intra-articular changes, osteochondrosis dissecans (OD), structural disorder, arthrosis, TU, dysostosis, and so on, for example in case of joint effusion of unclear genesis.

– Held X-ray stress recordings before secondary ligament reconstruction.

– Lack of adequate trauma.

– When an intra-articular cartilage/bone lesion or OD is suspected and, if necessary, CT/MRI.

1.8 Pitfalls:

– Calcaneus, talus, and tarsal fractures in areas not accessible in sonography.

– Additional shaft fractures or proximal lower leg fractures.

– Undisplaced epiphyseal plate injuries.

– Systemic diseases (e.g., osteogenesis imperfecta, M. Ollier, etc.) are not easy to get by sonography alone.

– Stability check recommended after completion of treatment.

– Strict attention must be paid to maintain the original cutting plane during the stress test.

– Counter tension of the patient can conceal band instability during the initial examination. Then repeat after a week.

1.9 Red flags:

– Severe pain, swelling, and/or restricted movement without evidence of a fracture, capsular ligament lesion, or soft tissue lesion (cave DD: infection, TU, nerve root lesion, somatoform reaction, etc.).

– Fracture without adequate trauma.

– Pre-traumatic complaints at this location.

– Refracture.

– Increasing complaints under therapy.

– Family history of relevant systemic diseases.

– Ankle or hindfoot pain with stress pain after 7 days.

1.10 Algorithm: Ankle/hind and metatarsal injury: lateral chain.

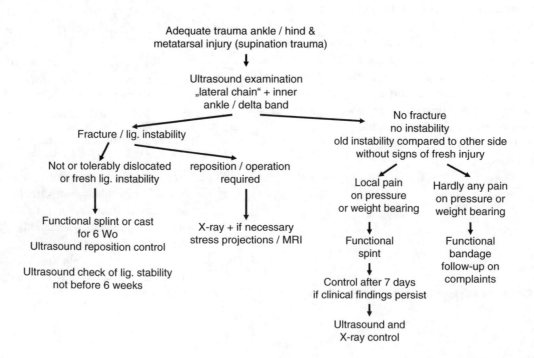

16.2 Introduction

The sprained ankle is the most common injury in sports, work, and leisure. Above all, the lateral bony and ligament structures of the distal lower leg, the upper and lower ankle, and the hind and metatarsus become affected. Functionally, these structures represent a "lateral chain" that can be checked sonographically for structural lesions and functional stability. Accidental injuries to the distal tibia, the inner ankle, the individual limbs of the delta ligament, and the dorsal hind and midfoot must also be excluded sonographically. The fractures to be observed after ankle distortion are mostly to be interpreted as bony ligament tears, except the fractures of the long bones and shear fractures during luxations. The ultrasound examination is free of radiation and pain and can be carried out easily and reliably after training and practice. Manual dexterity in sound head guidance and stress tests, as well as anatomical, spatial, and functional imagination is required for the examiner. After the initial clinical findings (deformity, swelling, hematoma, local pressure pain maximum, movement and stress pain, DMS) and evaluation, the standardized sonographic examination follows.

Historically, ultrasound for capsular ligament injuries of the ankle has a tradition of more than 30 years. Most authors have described sonography examination techniques with the aim of directly representing the structure of the respective volume in order to deduce its stability; this also applies to recent work [6]. Since the mid-1980s, various techniques have been described to partially stabilize the upper ankle joint (UAJ) using manually held stress to be measured from dorsal sectional planes [1–3] and information on the sensitivity and specificity of the respective technique compared to the X-ray findings and intraoperative findings. For the standardized examination technique shown here, the validity of the sonographic stability test on the outer ligaments and the anterior syndesmosis could be demonstrated, and orienting norm values were given in comparison with the X-rays and surgical findings [1]. Since then, this sonographic examination recommended by us has proven itself in daily practice and is carried out routinely after ankle and foot distortion [12–14]. Unfortunately, the sonographic examination techniques have not yet been adequately incorporated into the current radiological and orthopedic trauma surgery textbooks [19, 20]. This is justified by the resulting dependency of the examiner and nonuniform cutting planes and examination techniques. The MRI is considered the "golden standard" of the evidence of injury [5, 15, 16].

According to Ottawa Ankle Rules [11], part of the X-ray examinations can be dispensed with after ankle injuries. For forensic reasons, an X-ray standard image of the affected region in two planes (UAJ or rearfoot with metatarsus) is still recommended after sonographic clarification to document the position of fractures, to rule out incidental findings (e.g.

growth and buildup disorders, OD, tumor) and to document the bony status quo, the "current state" at the time of the examination. From an orthopedic point of view, the bone structure documents the previous skeletal and joint development and cannot be assessed sonographically in the same way.

16.3 Indication

After ankle, metatarsal, and metatarsal distortion, initial clinical examination and evaluation, ultrasound is indicated for the detection or exclusion of fresh capsular ligament injuries, instabilities, osseous ligament tears, and fractures regardless of age. If a primary fracture is suspected, it is recommended to take standard X-rays of the affected region in two planes before the sonographic examination in order to avoid unnecessary pain and an additional fragment dislocation during the sonographic stress tests. It is not uncommon for fractures which are not primarily recognized in the X-ray image to be determined sonographically. X-rays are essential for displaced long bones and intra-articular fractures. To assess the fragments and articular surfaces, further sectional imaging diagnostics may be necessary. Non-dislocated bony stress reactions without a cortical level and without a subperiosteal hematoma or reaction zone can only be detected on MRI as "bone bruise" (bone edema). On the uninjured ankle and foot, even in the subjectively symptom-free interval, if there is an appropriate question, the indication for the exclusion, or evidence of ligament instability is given, e.g. as part of an assessment.

A typical accident mechanism for structural injuries in the area of the lateral chain is the "stepping over" the ankle outward (supination trauma) [17, 18]. The ventral tibiofibular syndesmosis (VS) is particularly at risk when the foot rotates externally in dorsiflexion of the upper ankle, for example, with a rotational trauma in a closed ski boot. Dorsal tibiofibular syndesmosis (DS) is very vigorous and its isolated instability can rarely be visualized by sonography; in most cases, there is a bony tearing of the tibial origin, that is, of a dorsal Volkmann's triangle, which can be demonstrated from the dorsal as a contour step of the tibial cortex [19]. Sonographic evidence of a fresh instability of the VS, a fracture level of the dorsal tibia contour, or sonographic evidence of a lesion of the lig. fibulotalare posterius (FTP) or the DS, further radiological imaging is indicated [10–12].

A preliminary assessment of the expected structural injuries is already possible through the orientation clinical examination due to the localization of swelling, hematoma, and main pressure pain. In the area of the lateral chain, it is possible to "pull" all the links in the chain, but usually only one of the links breaks apart (discontinuity/

fracture). There are exceptions to multistage trauma, for example, primarily, a varus moment of stress acts on the upper ankle and then in a second step another stress impulse hits the lateral metatarsus or the MT5, or in the case of repeated trauma. Accidental injuries to neighboring regions, soft tissues, vessels, nerves, and tendons must be excluded clinically and, if necessary, sonographically, for example, of the peroneal tendons, tibialis anterior, and posterior tendons.

16.4 Contraindications and Indications for X-ray Diagnostics

In the case of open injuries, vascular or nerve injuries, the primary diagnosis and care in this regard is carried out; if necessary, also with a sectional image procedure, or, if necessary and available with qualification, with vascular or nerve sonography under hygienically perfect conditions. If displaced or displaceable fractures are detected, sonographic stress tests to check the ligament stability should be avoided in order not to endanger the fracture position and to avoid unnecessary pain.

If an operation is already clearly indicated based on the clinical examination, sonography can be dispensed with. Preoperative X-ray diagnosis is currently recommended for all planned operations, for documentation of the fracture position, for planning the procedure, in order not to overlook rare or accidental findings, and not least for forensic reasons.

If there is primarily no fracture, bony ligament rupture, or ligament instability to be demonstrated sonographically, at most a hypoechogenic soft tissue zone or a joint effusion, treatment is carried out using functional movement limitation using a bandage or U-splint and if symptoms persist, an ultrasound and X-ray check after 1 week. Individual patients are so tense during the initial examination that they cannot relax sufficiently during the sonographic stress tests. In the case of stress fractures of the distal fibula or metatarsal 5, a hypoechogenic periosteal reaction can be better demonstrated after 1 week. If there is sonographic evidence of effusion in the Chopart joint, a radiological examination of the tarsal bones, including the talus and calcaneus, is required at the appropriate clinic; if necessary with further diagnostic imaging.

We only recommend manual X-ray stress recordings to prove the instability of the FTA, FC, and VS in the case of old instabilities in the symptom-free interval preoperatively when the operation is requested to document the sonographically proven instability. Machine-held recordings, for example, B. with the device according to Scheuba, are obsolete because the patient's active counter tension cannot be taken into account.

16.5 Examination

Diagnostics and therapy follow the specified algorithm for injuries to the lateral chain. The anamnesis and the orientation clinical examination are followed by the sonographic examination. Simple, standardized positioning, sound head guidance with finger support on the patient, coupling of the probe "in the hanging drop" and dosed, sensitive examination technology allow a largely painless examination.

16.5.1 Positioning

The patient lies in a relaxed supine position, arms down, and he is asked to calm his stomach. Ergonomically best for patient and examiner is a height-adjustable couch, the examiner sits upright on a height-adjustable stool. A foot switch to freeze the sonography image is mandatory, as the examination requires both hands.

A wooden bench (approx. 14 cm edge length) or a comparable, noncompressible underlay is placed flat under the patient's lower leg, the ankle and the heel hang freely.

A roll or a second wooden bench under the knee prevents sagging and relaxes the lower leg muscles.

The examiner holds the upper ankle in the neutral 0 position. A 6 cm wide linear transducer with 7.5–12 MHz is ideal. It is sounded with plenty of gel "in a hanging drop," the little finger supported on the patient (Fig. 16.1).

16.5.2 Levels

The cutting planes for the "lateral chain" are (Fig. 16.2):

1. For the distal fibula, a longitudinal section from ventral, lateral, and dorsal (=semicircular).
2. For the ventral syndesmosis (VS), a cross-section from ventrally directly above the UAJ.
3. For the lig. fibulotalare anterius (FTA), a cross-section from ventrolateral over the neck of the talus.
4. For the lig. fibulocalcaneare (FC), longitudinal section over the course of the ligament.
5. Calcaneo cuboid joint (CC), a longitudinal section from lateral to dorsolateral.
6. Metatarsals 5 (MT5), a longitudinal section from dorsal, lateral, and plantar (=semicircular).

Further cutting levels:

y for the lig. fibulotalare posterius (FTP), a cross section from dorsolateral from the fibula to the talus.

z for dorsal syndesmosis (DS), a cross section from dorsolateral immediately above the UAJ.

Medial for the lig. deltoid (LD):

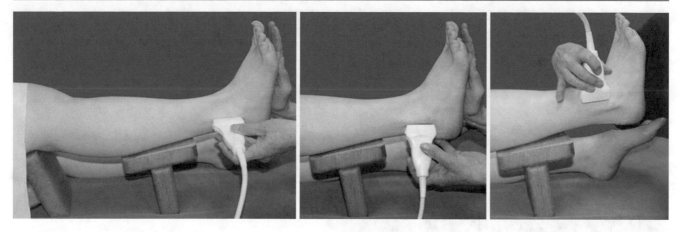

Fig. 16.1 Examination of ankle joint

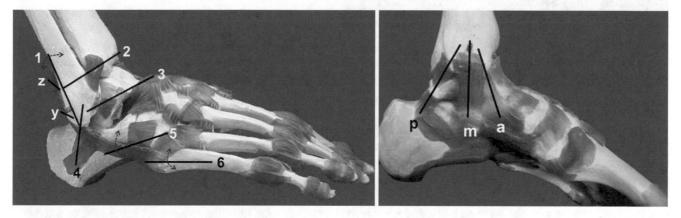

Fig. 16.2 Section planes for sonographic examination of injuries: Left in the area of the outer ligaments of the ankle and Chopart joint and the anterior syndesmosis ("lateral chain"). Right in the area of the inner ankle and over the three parts of the delta band (a pars tibiotalaris ant., m pars tibiocalcanearis, p pars tibiotalaris post)

p pars tibiotalaris posterior, longitudinal section over the dorsal part.

m pars tibiocalcanearis, longitudinal section over the middle part.

a pars tibiotalaris anterior, longitudinal section over the ventral part.

16.5.3 Setting

We start by examining the distal fibula (level 1), then metatarsal 5 (MT5) with the insertion of the peroneal tendons (level 6) to rule out fractures and bony ligament tears there. The contour of the respective bone is shown in a semicircular manner in longitudinal sections in a strictly vertical, sharp manner and examined for clear constant contour interruptions, contour steps, or periosteal elevations and hypoechogenic accompanying zones (Fig. 16.1). In the case of displaced fractures, the contour interruption and the fracture hematoma can hardly be overlooked. Fissures that are not or hardly displaced, stress fractures, or epiphyseal solutions require a subtle sonographic examination; if necessary also under metered manual stress and in the area of the main pressure pain (Fig. 16.3). If a metaphyseal periosteal elevation is discovered in comparison with the other side, it must be checked manually under sonographic observation whether it is a stress fracture without a cortex, an epiphyseal solution, or a co-reaction of the periosteum in the event of a syndesmosis or outer ligament injury. In the area of the trochlea peronealis, the distal fibula physiologically shows a small contour step without a subperiosteal reaction, which should not be confused with an infraction (Fig. 16.3). The sonographic assessment criteria for the detection of a fracture (Chapter Wrist 5.4) also apply here. It is advisable to check the integrity of the peroneal tendons in longitudinal and cross section for hypoechogenic accompanying zones, changes in anisotropy or caliber fluctuations, and subluxation in the same examination, as these are not infrequently involved [17]. At MT5 avulsion lesions of the peroneal apophysis, fractures, stress reactions and bony tears of the tendons and ligaments have to be differentiated.

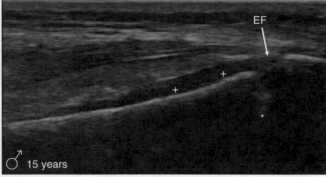

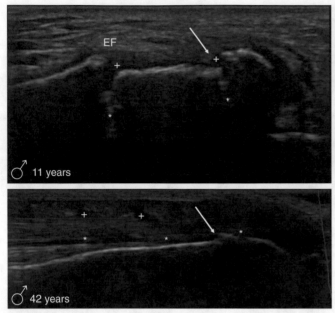

Fig. 16.3 Fibula distal longitudinal from lateral. Left ♂ 11 years, → demolition fracture of the fibula tip with the cortex, low hypoechogenic zone (HEZ+), and ring-down artifact (RdA*). Epiphyseal plate (EF) tolerant of pressure, cannot be dislocated. Right ♂ 15 years, metaphyseal periosteal lift (HEZ +) with local pressure tolerance proximal to the EF (→), no evidence of a cortex level, EF cannot be dislocated. Bottom: ♂ 42 years, physiological contour level at the retinaculum peronealis (→), no fracture! Section of the peroneal tendons (*), subcutaneous veins (+)

The front outer band, the lig. fibulotalare anterius (FTA), is most commonly affected in the supination trauma of the upper ankle. It is the "lanyard" for the lateral stability of the upper ankle and tensions between the FC and the FTP. It runs in a fan shape from the ventral distal fibula to the anterolateral talus and can only be shown in an unharmed manner in fan-shaped sections directly above the respective fiber course of the ligament, depending on the angle of incidence of the ultrasound, as an echogenic structure or, in the case of an oblique angle of incidence, as a hypoechogenic structure. However, the direct representation of the band structure alone does not allow a reliable statement on the stability of the band (Fig. 16.4); this requires a manual load test under standardized conditions in a cutting plane defined based on defined bony reference points [1, 8, 9, 12].

The leg is positioned as in Sect. 4.2. and shown in Fig. 16.5. The transverse cutting plane is precisely defined based on the bone contours (Fig. 16.2, level 3). It is located almost plantar parallel in the neutral-0 position from the ventral fibular edge over the talus neck to the os naviculare, has two contour peaks, and is identical to the neutral-0 position of the UAJ when the manual and ventral drawer in the UAJ is at rest and under stress [7]. Care must be taken to ensure that the original cutting plane is not lost during the stress test! A valid measurement is only possible if the measurement is carried out at rest and under load in the identical cutting plane.

After fresh trauma with local swelling and hematoma, the sonographic representability of the structural contours is usually better than in the uninjured state due to the increased fluid content in the tissue. An ultrasound gel pad can therefore be dispensed with. Hypoechogenic zones (HEZ) and local pressure pain indicate the location of the injured structures. A joint effusion is almost obligatory to prove in the event of an internal joint injury, fracture with joint involvement, capsular ligament lesion with instability, or activation of an OD or arthrosis as part of a distortion. If the outer ligaments and lateral capsule parts are severely torn, a joint effusion can flow into the soft tissues around the peroneal tendons and is then hardly detectable intra-articularly (Fig. 16.6). Swelling, HEZ, and joint effusion indicate a fresh ligament lesion in case of a verifiable ligament instability in the stress test. However, imaging alone does not distinguish with certainty a fresh ligament lesion from a redistortion with existing ligament instability. If the FTA is not injured, the change in distance is less than 2 mm, the measurement accuracy is ±1 mm. In the borderline case, the undamaged opposite side can be used for comparison. A side difference of >2 mm can be considered significant [1, 9, 12].

The specific question of pre-traumas that have occurred can often not be answered with certainty, much less the question of the type and duration of any pretreatment that has taken place and the extent of the stability that has been regained. After the treatment of a band instability has been completed, the sonographic examination of the achieved stability of the affected ligaments must be requested in order to be able to know the stability before the new trauma and to determine the necessary treatment in the case of a recurrent injury.

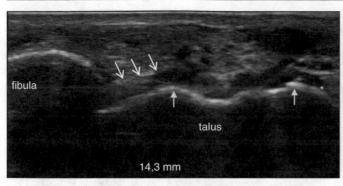
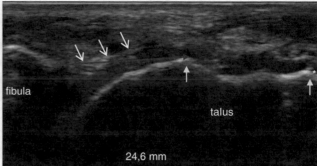

Fig. 16.4 ♂ 48 years, old FTA instability 3°: left neutral 14.3 mm distance of the fibula contour to the first talus peak (yellow arrow), right when stress is applied ventral talus drawer with an increase in the distance to 24.6 mm. The capsular ligament structures (↓↓↓) are echogenic but are not stable when subjected to stress. No joint effusion, at most a small hypoechogenic surrounding zone, that is, no indication of fresh soft tissue injury. (*) Talonavicular joint

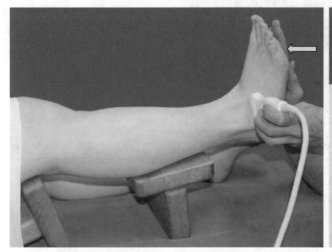
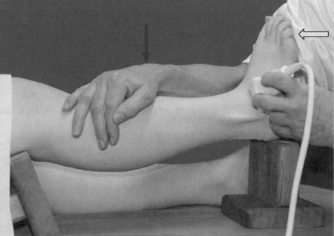

Fig. 16.5 Bearing for testing the FTA, UAJ held in neutral 0 position (yellow arrows): left at rest, heel free, lower leg underlaid. Stress on the right through the front drawer in the UAJ, heel underlaid, metered manual pressure on the lower leg dorsally (red arrows)

The ventral tibiofibular syndesmosis (VS), the lig. tibiofibular anterius, is next shown in the sagittal cross section immediately proximal to the upper ankle from obliquely ventrolateral (Fig. 16.2, level 2). The plane is slightly proximal to the cutting plane for the FTA. In the undamaged state, the VS can be depicted as a strong, echogenic band structure without a surrounding HEZ. After a strain (lesion 1°), the ligament structure of the VS is loosened hypoechogenically, possibly with a hypoechogenic accompanying zone, but without evidence of instability in the subsequent stress test. A step near the beginning or an interruption of the tibial or fibular bone contour with a ring-down artifact and/or fracture hematoma is an indication of a bony ligament tear and reason to carry out the stress test under ultrasound control with particular care and in order to be able to observe a movement of the fragment if necessary. The band structure shown at rest does not allow to judge its biomechanical stability sufficient enough. Any instability can only be demonstrated and measured using a standardized stress test [4].

For the stress test of the VS, the UAJ is initially in the rest and neutral 0 position immediately proximal to the UAJ (Fig. 16.7), and the bone distance between tibia and fibula or the width of the ring-down artifact between tibia and fibula is measured. Then, in the identical section plane with passive dorsal extension and external rotation in the UAJ, the image with the maximum achievable distance between tibia and fibula is frozen and the distance is measured again (Figs. 16.8, 16.9, 16.10, and 16.11 on the right). It is very important to ensure that the original cutting plane is not lost during the stress test! A valid measurement is only possible if the measurement is carried out at rest and under load in the identical cutting plane. If the VS is undamaged, the change in distance

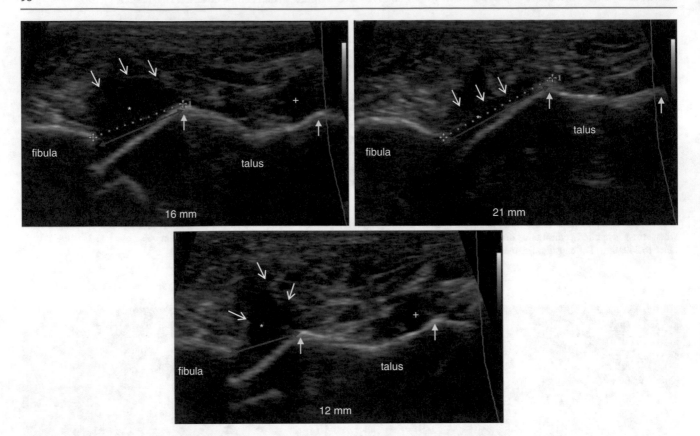

Fig. 16.6 ♂ 15 years, fresh FTA instability 3°: left neutral 16 mm distance of the fibula contour to the first talus peak (proximal yellow arrow), on the right when stressed ventral talus drawer with increasing the distance to 21 mm, no stop. The capsular ligament structures (↓↓↓) are thinly echogenic, neutral around the joint effusion (*) in the UAJ, not stable under stress, the joint effusion is distributed. At the bottom when extending the UAJ by maximum tension of the toe lifters, the fibulo-talar distance is reduced to 12 mm, the joint effusion (*) bulges more steeply. Notice the hypoechogenic environment also dorsally on the talonavicular joint (+)

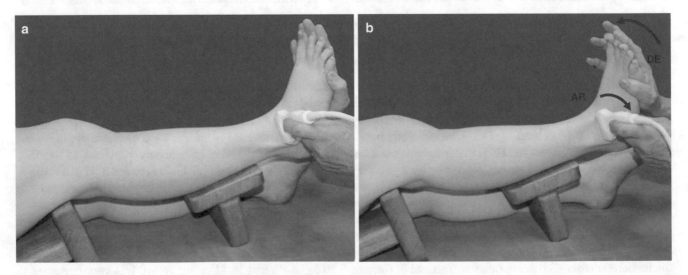

Fig. 16.7 Examination of the VS at rest (neutral position, left) and with maximum dorsiflexion (DE) and external rotation (AR) in the UAJ (right)

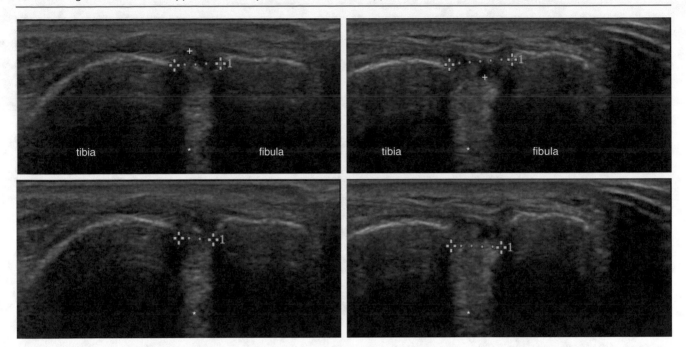

Fig. 16.8 VS stability test after old UAJ injury on the left, ♀ 60 years. Distance left tibia–fibula at rest (bone contour above 5.3 mm, width ring-down artifact (*) below 4.0 mm). Right distance tibia–fibula in stress in max. dorsal extension and external rotation (upper bone con-tour 7.4 mm, wide ring-down artifact * lower 5.9 mm), each >1 mm, that is, slight instability, lesion 2°, with low HEZ (+), which is drawn into the interosseous space when stressed

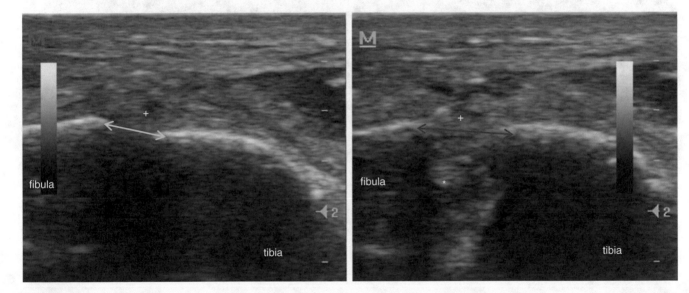

Fig. 16.9 VS stability test after a fresh injury to the right UAJ, ♂ 19 years. Bone contour distance fibula–tibia left 4.9 mm at rest, right with stress in max. dorsiflexion and external rotation 9.9 mm, differ-ence 5.0 mm = >4 mm without stop, that is, 3° lesion with HEZ (+). No ring-down artifact at rest (*)

is less than 1 mm, the measurement accuracy is ±1 mm. In the borderline case, the opposite side can be used for comparison [9, 12]. In order to stabilize the leg during external rotation, it is helpful if an auxiliary person fixes the tibia head of the patient firmly against rotation with both hands.

The middle outer band (FC), the lig. fibulocalcaneare, in supination trauma of the upper ankle, is usually only affected after or in addition to the injury to the FTA. It runs slightly fan-shaped from the tip of the fibula to the base of the tub. innominatum on the lateral calcaneus beneath the peroneal tendons, bridges two joints, the upper and lower ankle, and shows a greater latitude of the physiologically possible distance increase under manual stress during varus supination than VS and FTA. The ankle, heel, and foot must be freely

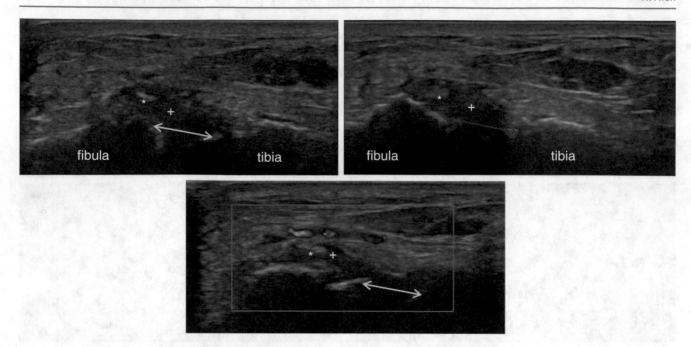

Fig. 16.10 Stability test after a fresh injury to the VS on the right, ♂ 57 years. Left bone contour distance fibula–tibia above at rest 4.4 mm. Right in case of stress in max. dorsal extension and external rotation 7.8 mm, difference 3.4 mm, that is, 2° lesion with clear HEZ (+), minimal bony tear (*). Bottom vessels

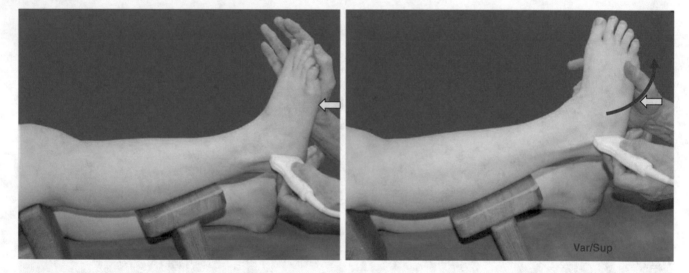

Fig. 16.11 Examination of the FC: left in a neutral position, right under varus/supination stress (Var/Sup). Loose counterpressure against spontaneous pointed foot position (yellow arrow)

supported for the examination (Fig. 16.11), the cutting plane for the FC follows the band course (Fig. 16.2, level 4).

The undamaged FC is scanned directly above the ligament from the side in a slight varus stress, depending on the angle of incidence, as a slight hypo- or hyperechogenic continuous structure below the cross section of the peroneal tendons. In the case of rupture of the FC, this continuous structure is missing; in the case of a fresh injury, an attempt is made to display the ligament directly. Usually there is a, a heteroechogenic hematoma zone around the peroneal ten-

dons, in which the FC rupture stumps are difficult to differentiate (Fig. 16.12). In the neutral position, the distance from the contour end of the fibula tip to the base of the tub. innominatum is now first measured and documented in the picture. Then a varus supination stress is exerted manually in the UAJ up to the pain limit in the identical section plane and the maximum achievable increase in distance is measured and documented in the image (Fig. 16.13). During varus stress, the sound probe and rearfoot must be moved together like a block opposite the fibula. It is very important to ensure that

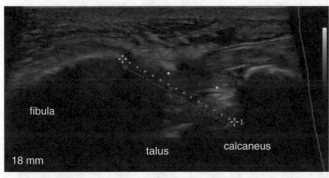

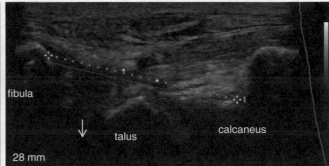

Fig. 16.12 FC stability test after a fresh injury to the UAJ on the left, ♂ 25 years. Left at rest, distance from bone contour of the fibula tip to the base of the tub. innominatum calcanei 18 mm, on the right with stress in max. varus/supination position of the UAJ 28 mm, difference

10 mm = > 4 mm without stop, that is, FC unstable 3° with HEZ in the area. Band structure of the FC cannot be delimited throughout, peroneal tendons (*) in cross section with HEZ. Ring-down artifact in the UAJ, yellow arrow

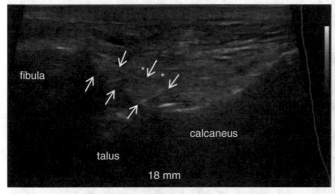

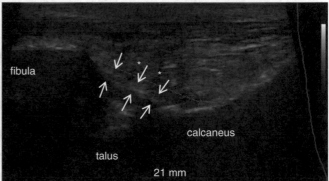

Fig. 16.13 FC stability test without fresh injury to the UAJ on the left, ♂ 45 years. Left at rest distance from the bone contour of the fibula tip-base tub. innominatum calcanei 18 mm, on the right with stress in max.

varus/supination position of the UAJ 21 mm, difference 3.0 mm = <4 mm with fixed stop, that is, FC stable without HEZ. White arrows delimit FC, Peroneus tendons (*) in cross section without HEZ

the original cutting plane is not lost during the stress test! A valid measurement is only possible if the measurement is carried out at rest and under load in the identical cutting plane. If the FC is not injured, the change in distance is less than 4 mm, the measurement accuracy is ±2 mm. In the borderline case, the undamaged opposite side can be used for comparison. In the case of complete FC instability, no stop and a ring-down artifact in the upper ankle joint can be observed in case of extreme varus stress (Fig. 16.12).

The dorsolateral Chopart ligament, the lig. calcaneocuboideum (CC), is often affected in supination–inversion trauma to the ankle and midfoot. The injury is often overlooked if you limit yourself to examining the ankle itself. Except for a two-stage or multistage trauma mostly either the FTA or the CC is ruptured and unstable, the other one pulled at best without loss of stability since both bands represent a chain together with the fibula and the MT5 in the case of varus supination inversion loading. The CC runs slightly fan-shaped from the dorsolateral calcaneus to the cuboid. The lateral parts of the ligament are tight and prevent lateral opening in the plantar plane. The dorsolateral

parts allow little mobility in the Chopart joint during supination. Small bony tears of the affected band parts can often be detected sonographically, but can only be shown in the X-ray image if they are projected at the edges [18]. The affected foot is stored freely for examination (Fig. 16.14), the cutting plane for the CC follows the course of the lateral and/or dorsolateral ligament portions semicircularly (Fig. 16.2, level 5).

Undamaged the CC is pictured directly above the respective ligament parts from lateral to dorsolateral as a hyperechogenic, continuous structure bridging the joint gap without surrounding HEZ. In the case of adduction stress, it is not possible to open it laterally in the plantar plane; in the case of supination loading, there is the physiologically little opening of the CC joint dorsolaterally. When straining the band parts without loss of stability, they are loosened, surrounded by a HEZ, and locally sensitive to pressure. In the event of rupture of the CC, increased lateral or dorsolateral opening ability under manual adduction or supination loading can also be demonstrated, depending on whether lateral or dorsolateral ligament portions or all are affected. In the case of osseous tear

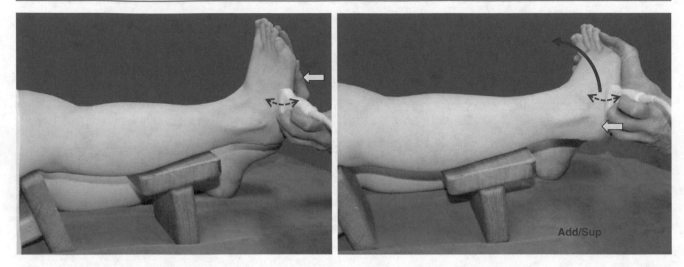

Fig. 16.14 Examination of the CC, scan the cutting plane semicircularly (<‒‒‒>): left in a calm neutral position, right under adduction and or supination stress (Add/Sup). Loose counterpressure against the spontaneous pointed foot and the calcaneus (yellow arrow)

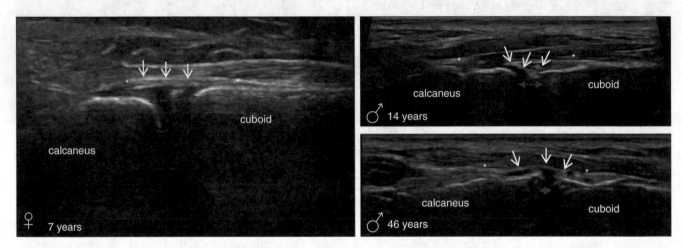

Fig. 16.15 CC band uninjured: left ♀ 7 years, top right ♂ 14 years, bottom right ♂ 46 years. White arrows mark the band structures, red double arrow the sono-graphic joint gap. No abnormal HEZ, incisions of the peroneal tendons (*)

fractures, the dislocability of the fragment can be observed sonographically in the stress test. A joint effusion in the Chopart joint that persists for more than a week can be an indication of an internal joint injury in the lower ankle and should then be clarified with further imaging diagnostics, if necessary also with a sectional image procedure. In the case of CC injuries, the possible involvement of the peroneal tendons in the immediate vicinity up to the approach on the MT 5 can also be excluded sonographically. A numerical measurement of the sonographically verifiable instability has so far not proven itself, since the band parts affected differently do not allow a sensible standardization of the instability, and differentiated therapeutic consequences have not yet been drawn from it. The isolated fresh CC instability is treated by consistent functional splinting for 4–6 weeks under load up to the pain limit, for example, in the ready-made shoe, and thereby the safe exclusion of a redistortion (Figs. 16.15 and 16.16).

Dorsal tibiofibular syndesmosis (DS), the lig. tibiofibulare posterius, is checked if there is an instability of the ventral syndesmosis (VS). The DS is shown in the sagittal cross section immediately proximal to the upper ankle from obliquely dorsolateral (Fig. 16.2 level z, Fig. 16.17). Between the Achilles tendon and the Peroneus tendons, the DS is shown in the uninjured state as a strong, continuous, echogenic band structure without a surrounding HEZ. After a strain (lesion 1°), the ligament structure of the VS is loosened hypoechogenically, possibly with a hypoechogenic accompanying zone. With the relatively rare partial or complete rupture, the detection of a consistently echogenic ligament structure by hematoma is difficult or no longer possible. A validated manual stress test to measure the stability of the DS has not been published to date and cannot be recommended without further exclusion of additional osteochondral lesions in the ankle area through further imaging. A step

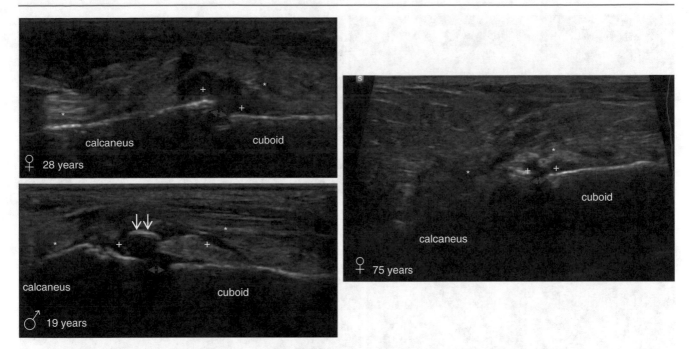

Fig. 16.16 CC ligament after injury: top left ♀ 28 years fresh ligament rupture with HEZ (+) and effusion. Bottom left ♂ 19 years with fresh bony ligament tear (↓↓). Top right ♀ 75 years, 3-week-old ligament injury with residual HEZ without joint effusion. Incisions of the peroneal tendons (*)

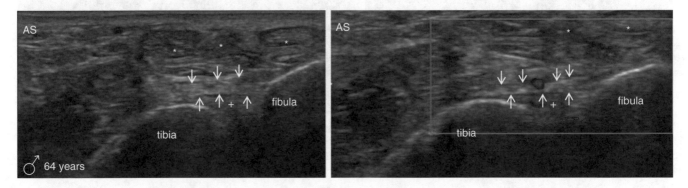

Fig. 16.17 Cross section over the intact dorsal tibiofibular syndesmosis (DS): Between the white arrows superficial, vertically struck parts of the band, including deep, somewhat obliquely struck parts of the band (+). Incisions of the peroneal tendons (*). Distance between tibia and fibula (RdA, red double arrow). The cross section of the Achilles tendon (AS) is just outside the image section at the top left. Right blue A. peronaea

near the beginning or interruption of the tibial or fibular bone contour with a ring-down artifact and/or fracture hematoma is an indication of a bony ligament tear.

The rear outer band (FTP), the lig. fibulotalare posterius, is rarely affected in supination trauma of the upper ankle, at most after the previous rupture of the FTP and FC or with atypical, varus impulse loading in dorsiflexion of the UAJ with thrust loading on the calcaneus and talus from dorsal. The isolated ligament rupture is less common than the fibular bony ligament tear. The FTP is to be shown unharmed in the transverse section from dorsolateral directly above the course of the band with a vertical sound incidence as a strong, echogenic band structure, with oblique sound incidence slightly hypoechogenic without conspicuous hypoechogenic accom-

panying zone (Fig. 16.18). If this ligament structure is loosened after trauma (strain, 1° lesion) or if the continuity of the ligament structure between the fibula and talus cannot be demonstrated with manual doses, a partial or complete lesion (2° or 3°) can be assumed. A validated manual stress test to measure stability has not yet been described for FTP, the significance of the injury and the further diagnostic and therapeutic consequences required depend on the additional injuries that may be present. The demonstrably isolated injury can consistently be treated conservatively with a functional splint and/or circular stabilizing bandage with good results, such as the FTA.

Due to the similar clinical symptoms in the injury, sonographic clarification also requires a lengthwise sec-

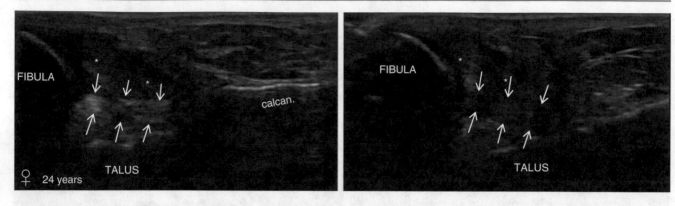

Fig. 16.18 Cross section over the uninjured lig. fibulotalare posterius (FTP): FTP echogenic between the white arrows on the left, hypoechogenic hit slightly obliquely on the right. Incisions of the peroneal tendons (*)

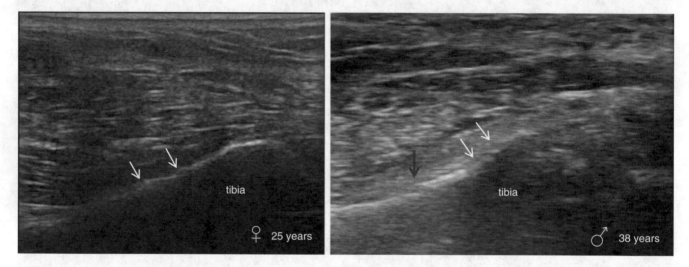

Fig. 16.19 Longitudinal section from dorsal over the distal tibia: On the left no pathological level of the bone contour, but artificial contour disturbances due to geometric distortions of the sonopicture due to the fibrous-like septa of the soft tissues in front (white arrows). On the right, clearly pathological contour level (red arrow) in Volkmann fracture, which can easily be missed in the lateral X-ray image

tion over the dorsal tibia to be carefully searched for a fracture level, as an indication of a possible Volkmann fracture of the dorsal tibial joint surface (Fig. 16.19). Sonographic diagnostics require a subtle and careful examination of the dorsal, lateral, and medial tibia contour in longitudinal sections.

A fracture of the inner ankle, the malleolus medialis tibiae, and a lesion of the delta ligament (LD), the lig. deltoideum, can also primarily be excluded sonographically after ankle distortion with additional medial clinical symptoms [7]. First, a fracture is ruled out in semicircular longitudinal sections above the inner ankle from medial, ventral, and dorsal. The structure continuity of the anterior, middle, and dorsal part of the delta band follows.

Medially, the talus is guided through the inner ankle, mainly bony, reinforced by the strong delta band. Isolated ruptures of the delta ligament are therefore rare; usually, there is a fracture of the inner ankle or individual parts of the ligament rupture in connection with fractures of the outer ankle or ruptures of the outer ligaments. The sonographic examination and measurement of the stability of the delta band using a manual stress test has so far not proven itself. Isolated lesions of individual parts of the delta band can be healed conservatively with functional splinting.

16.5.4 Assessment

Fractures of the fibula, the MT5, the tibia, the inner ankle, and bony ligament tears are to be addressed according to the criteria assessed above and, if necessary, documented radiologically, splinted and, if necessary, reduced or provided with operative care (Figs. 16.3, 16.20, 16.21).

An isolated injury of VS, FTA, FC, and CC with a hypoechoic loosened ligament structure and surrounding zone without fracture and without instability proof only requires functional splinting and protection to the strain (lesion 1°) to allow painless mobility and resilience.

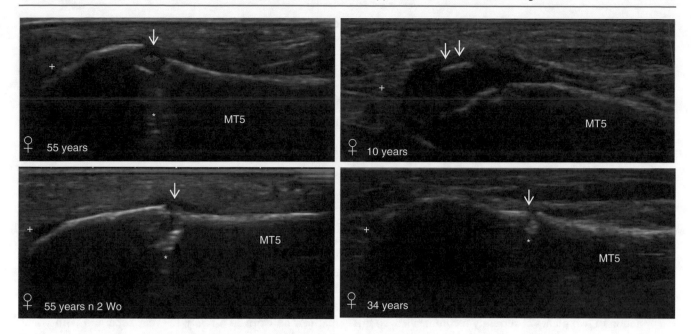

Fig. 16.20 MT5 longitudinally from lateral: Left ♀ 55 years, (↓) demolition fracture MT5 base with the cortex, (↔) fracture gap, fresh on top, below after 2 weeks. Top right ♀ 10 years, apophyseal nucleus (os vesalii ↓↓) with hypoechogenic, hyaline cartilaginous surrounding zone without signs of injury. Bottom right ♀ 34 years Johnson stress fracture (↓) after excessive jogging. Ring-down artifact (RdA*), attachment of the peroneal tendon (+)

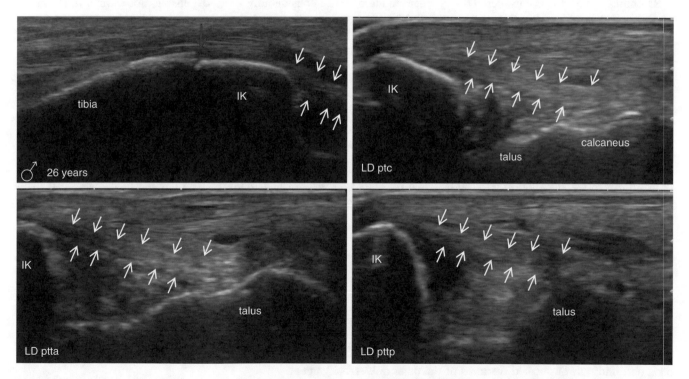

Fig. 16.21 Malleolus medialis tibiae (inner ankle, IK) and lig. deltoid (LD): top left ♂ 26 years transverse fracture of the inner ankle (red arrow). Upper right LD middle part, pars tibiocalcanearis (ptc) intact. Lower left LD ventral part, pars tibiotalaris ant. (ptta) and lower right dorsal part, pars tibiotalaris post. (pttp) each intact

If, in addition to the fresh injury signs of the VS, a relevant instability of 2–4 mm or a non- or <1 mm dislocated bone tear in the ultrasound is demonstrated (lesion 2°, partial lesion), a decision must be made using standard X-rays to determine whether conservative treatment with a functional splint/orthosis is possible, or whether surgical stabilization is advisable. In the event of fresh instability of the VS of >4 mm, osseous tear with a dislocation of >1 mm (3° lesion, complete lesion), significant joint effusion, and possibly further structural injuries, further diagnostics to clarify the surgical indication are indicated.

16.5.5 Diagnosis

The diagnosis is made sonographically and if there is an intolerable position of any bony fragments or ligament lesions 2° (partial instability) or 3° (complete instability), an X-ray examination in two planes is currently recommended, so that no additional injuries or incidental findings with possibly special therapy options can be overlooked. If necessary, sonographically proven instability can be documented and verified preoperatively using manually held special X-rays.

The previous comparative studies mostly relate to the MRI findings; the MRI is considered the "golden standard" of injury detection on the ligament, bone, and cartilage structures due to the increased water or proton content there. However, the extent of instability is not measurable in the standard MRI, but only with limited sensitivity through manually held X-rays under stress or through intraoperative measurements. At best, the stability of capsular and ligament structures can be inferred indirectly on MRI. Using manual stress tests in the standardized sonographic techniques described, the stability of the band structure in question can be directly demonstrated in vivo with little effort and radiation-free, and can be measured reproducibly. The examination is almost painless and can be repeated as required. It has proven itself to us as the "golden standard" of proof of stability or instability even after old injuries.

16.5.6 Therapy and Controls

The therapy is based on the current guidelines for the treatment of existing bony or ligamentous injuries to the ankle, back and midfoot. Dislocated fractures of the outer ankles, type Weber B and C, require further radiological diagnostics for therapy decisions or preoperatively. Slightly dislocated, isolated fibular fractures type Weber B and A with a sonographic cortical level of <1 mm on all sides can be treated conservatively with a functional splint or functional circular cast bandage, as well as fresh lesions 1° and 2° of the VS, the ankle outer ligaments (FTA and FC), the ligaments of the

dorsolateral Chopart joints (CC) and not or only sightly displaced tearing fractures of the MT5 base, after the patient has been informed about the treatment options and has given his consent. Before a primary surgical treatment in the case of a fresh rupture of the FC and a fresh demolition fracture of the base of the MT5, the advantages and disadvantages and the treatment options in the specific case must be discussed with the patient concerned. The patient is then left with the final decision as to whether surgical or conservative treatment is desired.

After completing the primary clinical and sonographic diagnostics and any necessary standard X-rays, stabilization in a functional lower leg UAJ-U splint is recommended; if necessary with heel inclusion in the event of a lesion of the FTA or with the inclusion of the midfoot in the event of a lesion of the CC or tearing fracture of the MT5 Base. After 1–2 weeks of swelling, the splint is replaced for a further 3 weeks with a functional, circular cast bandage that can be worn in a ready-to-wear shoe and with which stress and movement up to the pain limit are permitted. After the circular bandage has been removed, the original U-splint must be worn again in the ready-made lace-up shoe until the end of the sixth week after the injury [12]. Assembled splints and orthoses are used alternatively, but are considerably more expensive, not always functionally equivalent, and do not ensure patient compliance to the same extent.

Checks are carried out as required or after 1 week, in the case of fractures sonography or X-ray, in the case of ligament instabilities, the stability is only checked after the end of treatment, at the earliest after 6 weeks and at the latest before the next injury. The ultrasound stability control after healing is necessary. It is the only way to decide after a new injury, whether there is a preexisting residual instability in the case of a pre-injury that is not fully healed, or a new fresh lesion if the ligament has healed stably. If there are clear clinical signs of a fresh injury, excluded bony injury, and initially no evidence of ligament instability in the sonogram, the sonographic stability test should be repeated after 1 week at the latest in order to demonstrate an instability that, in rare cases, could not initially be detected in primarily very tense patients. After the first and before the sixth week of treatment, a sonographic stability test should be avoided in the case of fresh ligament lesions in order not to disrupt the healing process during the necessary consequent functional immobilization of the damaged ligament.

16.6 Pitfalls and Red Flags

In the case of skin abrasions, open wounds, and extensive soft tissue injuries, caution is necessary to avoid unnecessary pain, the hygiene regulations must be observed and infections can be excluded. In the case of open fractures and dislocations with soft tissue injuries, nerve and/or vascular injuries in the foreground, the treatment of these injuries has priority over sonography.

A post-traumatic sonographically clearly identifiable joint effusion in the ankle or Chopart joint with clinical complaints without evidence of a fracture or capsular ligament injury requires further differential diagnosis and imaging, since it can be an internal joint injury that is not accessible to sonography (cartilage flake, OD, or the like) or a rheumatoid reaction, crystal arthropathy, activated arthrosis, and so on. This is especially true if effusion and discomfort persist for more than a week. Individual patients cannot relax easily during the initial examination, which is easy for the attentive examiner to perceive. In these cases it is recommended to perform or repeat the sonographic stress test of the band in question well dosed and carefully after a week of immobilization in a functional splint if there is a sign of a not or only slightly displaced fracture or epiphyseal solution, and if this is necessary for the diagnosis and therapy decision (see above).

Prevention of thrombosis is obligatory by applying functionally correct splints and adequate bandages with sufficient compression and by instructing the patient to rest with the legs elevated, to do foot exercises in order to reduce venous stasis, and to try to make ground contact with the foot and put weight on it up to the pain limit while walking with or without walker, if possible. Under these conditions and after explanation and their informed consent, most patients with ambulatory treatable injuries of the AS or the outer ligaments can do without anticoagulant drug prophylaxis, which can be limited to high risk patients.

When pain increases and the patient complains, bandages and splints must be checked immediately for tightness and pressure marks, and signs of circulation problems, thrombosis, and sensomotoric deficits must be excluded. If any of these complications turn up, they require an immediate solution and have to be further diagnosed and treated accordingly.

References

Comparative Examination X-ray/Sonography/Surgical Findings/MRI

1. Schricker T, Hien NM, Wirth CJ. Klinische Ergebnisse sonographischer Funktionsuntersuchungen der Kapselbandläsionen am Knie—und Sprunggelenk. Ultraschall. 1987;8:27–31.
2. Glaser F, Friedl W, Welk E. The value of ultrasound in the diagnosis of capsule ligament injuries of the upper ankle joint. Unfallchirurg. 1989;92:540–6.
3. Ernst R, Grifka J, Gritzan R, Kemen M, Weber A. Sonographische Kontrolle des Außenbandapparates am oberen Sprunggelenk bei der frischen Bandruptur und chronischen Bandinstabilität. Z Orthop. 1990;128:525–30.
4. Oae K, Takao M, Naito K, Uchio Y, Kono T, Ishida J, et al. Injury of the tibiofibular syndesmosis: value of MR imaging for diagnosis. Radiology. 2003;227:155–61.
5. Joshy S, Abdulkadir U, Chaganti S, Sullivan B, Hari- haran K. Accuracy of MRI scan in the diagnosis of ligamentous and chondral pathology in the ankle. Foot Ankle Surg. 2010;16:78–80.
6. Cheng Y, Cai Y, Wang Y. Value of ultrasonography for detecting chronic injury of the lateral ligaments of the ankle joint compared with ultrasonography findings. Br J Radiol. 2014;87:20130406.
7. Lechner R, Richter H, Friemert B, Palm HG, Gottschalk A. Vergleich der Sonografie und der Magnetresonanz-tomografie zur Diagnostik von Rupturen des Lig. deltoideum—gibt es einen Unterschied? Z Orthop Unfall. 2015;153:408–14.

Textbook Contributions Sonography Ligament Injuries/Instability Ankle and Foot

8. Hien NM. Stabilitätsprüfung Sprunggelenk. In: Graf R, Schuler P (Hrsg.) Sonographie am Stütz- und Bewegungsapparat bei Erwachsenen und Kindern. Lehrbuch und Atlas, 2. Auflage. Weinheim: VCH; 1995. p. 297–308.
9. Hien NM. OSG-Instabilität. In: Gaulrapp H, Szeimies U (Hrsg). Diagnostik der Gelenke und Weichteile. Sonographie oder MRT. Elsevier: Munich; 2008. p. 195–197.
10. Stäbler A, Szeimies U, Walther M. Bildgebende Diagnostik des Fußes. Stuttgart: Thieme; 2013. p. S34–7.

Diagnostic and Treatment Concepts, Review Articles

11. Stiell IG, McKnight RD, Greenberg GH, McDowell I, Nair RC, Wells GA, Johns C, Worthington JR. Implementation of the Ottawa ankle rules. JAMA. 1994;271(11):827–32.
12. Hien NM. Ein praxisnahes, effektives Behandlungskonzept bei Kapselbandverletzungen des oberen Sprunggelenkes und Mittelfußes aufgrund sonografischer Differenzierung. Orthop Prax. 2002;38(7):489–94.
13. Gaulrapp H. Funktionelle sonografische Diagnostik bei Kapsel-Band-Verletzungen am OSG. Trauma Berufskrankh. 2015;17:15–21.
14. Gaulrapp H, Lins S, Walther M. Möglichkeiten der funktionellen sonografischen Diagnostik bei der Primärbehandlung fibularer Kapsel-Band-Verletzungen des Sprunggelenks. FussSprungg. 2016;14:137–45.
15. Harrasser N, Eichelberg K, Pohlig F, Waizy H, Toepfer A, von Eisenhart-Rothe R. Laterale Instabilität des oberen Sprunggelenks. Orthopäde. 2016;45(11):1001–14.
16. Hank C. Von der Außenbandruptur zur chronischen Instabilität. OUP. 2017;7(8):396–400.
17. Klos K, Knobe M, Randt T, Simons P, Mückley T. Verletzungen der Peronealsehnen. Häufig übersehen. Unfallchirurg. 2017; 120:1020–30.

Anatomical and Biomechanical Basics

18. Zobel K. Das unerkannte Adduktionstrauma im Calcaneo-Cuboid-Gebiet: Die häufigste Fußwurzel-Vorfuß-Verletzung.

Ihre Sichtbarmachung im Röntgenbild. Z Orthop Ihre Grenzgeb. 1969;104(4):806–16.

19. Bohndorf K, et al. Akutes Trauma und Überlastung, Sprunggelenk und Fuß. In: Radiologische Diagnostik der Knochen und Gelenke (2). Stuttgart: Thieme; 2014. p. 224–47.

20. Vetter S, Grützner P. Bandverletzungen am oberen Sprunggelenk. In: Wirth CJ, Mutschler W, Kohn D, Pohlemann T, editors. Praxis der Orthopädie und Unfallchirurgie. Stuttgart: Thieme; 2014. p. 846–55.

Further Reading

21. Wirth CJ, Artmann M. Chronische fibulare Sprunggelenksinstabilität—Untersuchungen zur Röntgendiagnostik und Bandplastik. Arch Orthop Unfallchir. 1977;88:313–20.

Fractures of Fifth Metatarsal

Ole Ackermann

17.1 Synopsis

1.1 Rationale of application: position control, detection/exclusion of a dislocation.
1.2 Evidence level: IV.
1.3 Indication: conservative treatment for radiologically proven MFK 5 base fracture.
1.4 Contraindications: after plate osteosynthesis.
1.5 Age of the patient: any age.
1.6 Examination: longitudinal section in three planes: MFK 5 base from dorsal, lateral, and plantar.
1.7 Indications for additional X-ray diagnostics: suspected dislocation.
1.8 Pitfalls: slow dislocation.
1.9 Red flags: persistent pain.
1.10 Fig. 17.1 Follow-up SAFE algorithm, adapted for MFK 5 basis (see also Chap. 5.2).

17.2 Introduction

Treatment of a secured base fracture of the fifth metatarsal is based on dislocation and stability. If no primary relevant shift is evident, conservative treatment can be initiated. Position controls are important to ensure that dislocation is not overlooked. If such is diagnosed, surgical stabilization should take place.

The decisive factor here is the assessment of the fracture gap; in the event of instability, the fragments diverge further and the fracture gap becomes larger. This can be displayed quickly and easily using sonography. This speeds up the examination process and prevents radiation exposure.

17.3 Indication Including Patient Age

If an MFK basic fracture has been diagnosed and the decision to use conservative therapy has been made, the indication for ultrasound checks is given. The bone can be easily visualized using sonography and the width of the fracture gap can be measured.

Since no blinded studies have yet been published on this indication, exact information on the safety of the method compared to the X-ray display is not available. However, the good visualization of the structures and the simple technology make it very likely that the display will achieve a comparable or better quality than the conventional X-ray image.

17.4 Contraindications and Indications for X-ray Diagnostics

In the case of fractures treated with surgery, the fracture gap can also be assessed if a screw or wire/cerclage osteosynthesis has been carried out (in the case of plate restoration, this prevents the display in at least one, often even in two planes), the main disadvantage of sonography is, however, that a dislocation of the osteosynthesis material cannot be shown with certainty. Therefore, operative care is not a good indication for a sonographic position check at this time.

Whenever there is suspicion of dislocation, this should be confirmed radiologically. Although the X-ray usually does not provide any significant further findings, at the current level of evidence an operative revision without prior X-ray imaging appears to be problematic from a medical and medical–legal point of view.

O. Ackermann (✉)
Department of Orthopedic Surgery, Ruhr-University Bochum,
Bochum, Germany

© Springer Nature Switzerland AG 2021
O. Ackermann (ed.), *Fracture Sonography*, https://doi.org/10.1007/978-3-030-63839-9_17

Fig. 17.1 Follow-up SAFE from Chap. 5.1, applied to the MFK 5 basic fracture. (©Ole Ackermann 2020)

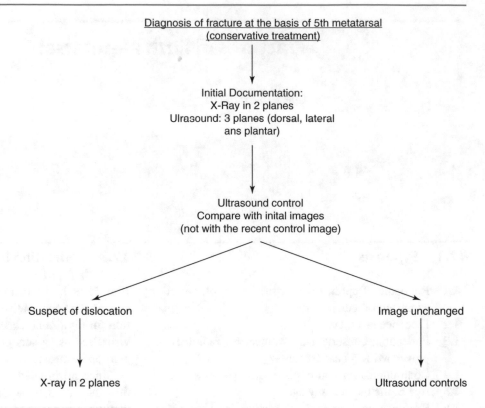

17.5 Examination

17.5.1 Positioning

The examination is done lying down with the linear transducer.

17.5.2 Levels

Three longitudinal planes are made: dorsal, lateral, and plantar.

17.5.3 Setting

After finding the bone, the transducer is positioned so that the cortex of the fifth MFK is shown across the entire width of the screen; if the image section is wider than the bone, the entire bone should be visible; this ensures the correct longitudinal cut.

The image section should capture the entire base proximally (Fig. 17.1).

17.5.4 Assessment

The typical aspect of a fracture with an interruption of the cortex is shown. Ultrasound can be used to visualize discrete, undislocated fractions (Fig. 17.2a–d). The width of the joint gap is measured and used for later comparison.

It is very important that the current examination is always compared with the first picture of the day of the accident, so as not to overlook a slow dislocation. The comparison is always made with the same level in the previous finding because the width of the fracture gap can be different in the three levels (Fig. 17.3a–e).

If an illustration is not possible, an X-ray check is carried out.

17.5.5 Diagnosis

The diagnosis of dislocation is made by directly comparing the width of the fracture gap.

17.5.6 Therapy and Controls

The number and frequency of the controls are individually determined by the practitioner; they should take place at the same intervals in which X-ray checks would also be indicated. Sonography can also be used to assess callus formation.

17.6 Pitfalls and Red Flags

Slow dislocations must not be overlooked in the examination, therefore, the first available sonograph finding (mostly from the day of the accident) is always used for comparison.

The joint gap width should also always be compared on the same ultrasound level, since there may also be differ-

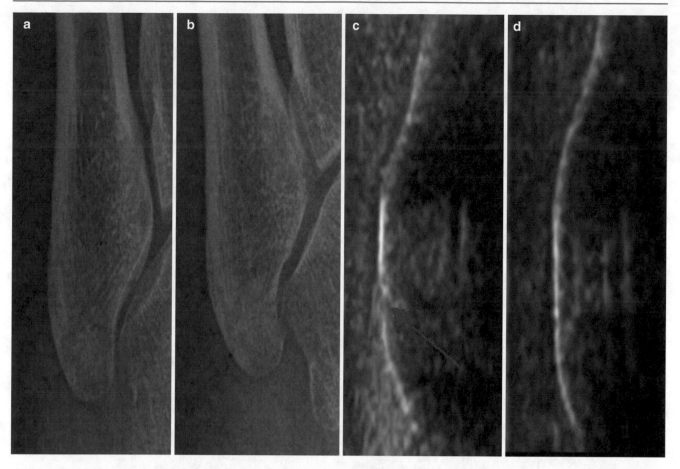

Fig. 17.2 Discrete undislocated fracture of the MFK 5 base. (**a, b**) X-ray image of the fracture, (**c, d**) sonographic imaging from dorsal and lateral. Red arrow: fracture. (©Ackermann and Eckert 2015; Courtesy of off label media)

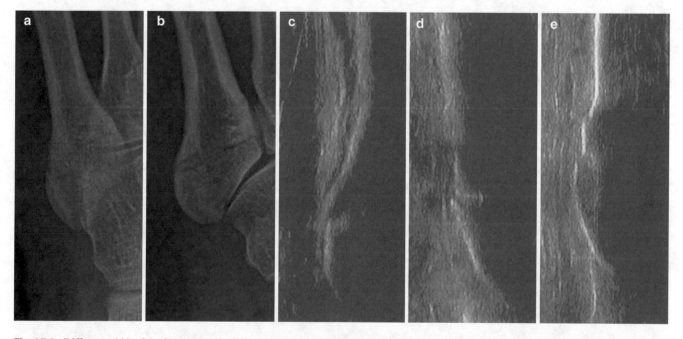

Fig. 17.3 Different width of the fracture gap in different planes. (**a, b**) X-ray image of the fracture, (**c–e**) sonographic imaging from dorsal, lateral, and plantar. (©Ackermann and Eckert 2015; Courtesy of off label media)

ences in the different levels. Standardization of the examination process and complete documentation are important here.

Increasing pain, swelling, and increasing stress insufficiency are always a reason for X-ray control.

Fractures of the Foot

Hartmut Gaulrapp

18.1 Synopsis

1.1 Rationale of application: X-ray free diagnosis and therapy of metatarsal fractures.

1.2 Evidence level: IIa.

1.3 Indication: screening to exclude an osseous injury after sprains and contusions of the hind- and middle foot, unclear foot pain in toddlers.

1.4 Contraindications: open fractures, visible malposition.

1.5 Age of the patient: all ages.

1.6 Examination: sonographic examination at the locus dolendi. At the distal fibula in the fibular and anterior longitudinal section. Screening of lateral ligaments (LTFA, LFTA, LFC, CC Ligament), longitudinal section over painful metatarsal bone, sagittally from anterior and plantar, and coronal from medial (metatarsal 1) or lateral (metatarsal 5), including the toe joints.

1.7 Indications for additional X-ray diagnostics:
   – sonographic suspicion of osseous injury.
   – persistent pain after 7 days if no fracture has been demonstrated.
   – planned surgery.
   – uncertainty in the assessment.
   – recurrent fractures.
   – positive history of pathologic bone metabolism, osteoporosis, or previously known stress fractures.

1.8 Pitfalls:
   – complex trauma.
   – joint injuries/joint instabilities.
   – pure internal bone lesions.
   – systemic diseases (e.g., osteogenesis imperfecta).

1.9 Red flags:
   – severe pain/immobility without proof of fracture.
   – fracture without adequate trauma.
   – pre-traumatic complaints at this location.
   – recurrent fractures.
   – increasing complaints under therapy.
   – family history of relevant systemic diseases.
   – persistent pain after 7 days.

H. Gaulrapp (✉)
Facharztpraxis für Orthopädie, Kinder-Orthopädie und Sportmedizin, München, Germany

18.2 Introduction

Lower limb injuries have their highest incidence in hind and midfoot. Inversion/supination injuries are the most common indirect contusions among the most common direct injury mechanism. At the ankle, the lateral malleolus is most often affected by fractures. Fractures on the foot in adolescents or adults mostly affect the base of the metatarsal 5. Stepping on a foot sometimes leads to isolated fractures of the metatarsals 2–4, while rollover or crush injuries can injure all metatarsals. Infants are most often injured at the base of metatarsal 1. Unclear pain syndromes on the metatarsus, less often on the rear foot, especially after a previous overload when running can indicate a stress fracture. Toe fractures are common, mostly banal, injuries.

18.3 Indication

If the patient's medical history and clinical diagnostics indicate that the malleoli or metatarsal bones are involved, imaging by ultrasound is carried out directly on the examination table. The toe bones and the tarsal bones are usually not indications for primary sonographic examination.

18.4 Contraindications and Indications for X-ray Diagnostics

Open injuries and typical signs of fracture, especially malpositions, are an indication for primary X-ray diagnosis.

18.5 Examination

18.5.1 Patients Positioning

The patient lies or sits on the examination table. The best way to examine the ankle is to support the knee with a roller and heel, and the foot with the plantar sole set on the table. The affected ankles or metatarsus´ locus dolendi is then located using the transducer.

© Springer Nature Switzerland AG 2021
O. Ackermann (ed.), *Fracture Sonography*, https://doi.org/10.1007/978-3-030-63839-9_18

18.5.2 Section Levels

The sonographic examination is performed on the distal fibula in the fibular and anterior longitudinal section. For the LTFA, LFTA, LFC, and CC joint sections please refer to the corresponding chapter. On the midfoot, the sagittal longitudinal section is performed from anterior and plantar as well as, due to anatomical reasons, only possible for the metatarsals 1 and 5, in coronary stratification, for the metatarsus 1 from the medial side, for the metatarsal bone 5 from the lateral side. The scanning starts from the Lisfranc joint row distally to the basic toe joint.

18.5.3 Setting

In the area of the distal fibula as well as the metatarsal bones there is only little subcutaneous tissue so that the sharp echogenic line of the bony surface with its dorsal sound extinction sometimes lies within the unfavorable near focus area. In children, the periosteum can be detected as a lower echogenic line, additionally the growth plates can be seen. At the base of the fifth metatarsal in a growing child, an apophysis can be seen not be confused with fractures (Fig. 18.1a, b). The apophysis runs almost parallel to the metatarsal bone, while fractures are usually perpendicular to it.

In principle, the attached joints are to be examined when examining adjacent bones. Tendons inserting on the bones, such as the short peroneal tendon at the fifth metatarsal bone should also be clarified.

18.5.4 Assessment

In children bruises sometimes lead to a pronounced periosteal hematoma, which can be seen as a bulge less hypoechoic line under the periosteum (Fig. 18.2). Fractures appear as an interruption of the echogenic bone line (Fig. 18.3a, b), mostly subcapital on the metatarsal bones 2–4 (Fig. 18.4). Kinking rarely occurs. The adjacent joints can be filled with an hypoechoic hemarthrosis. Salter Harris 1 injuries are rare (Fig. 18.5).

The assessment of injuries to the base of the first metatarsal bone in infancy is more difficult due to the broad almost echo-free hyaline cartilage, since local hemarthrosis formation sonographically is just as impressive. Fractures occurring at the base of the fifth metatarsal bone are divided into transverse (Fig. 18.6) or avulsion injuries (Fig. 18.7). The insertion of the usually uninjured short peroneal tendon can be safely assessed sonographically. Dislocations visible after 5 days are an indication for surgery. The Lisfranc injury at the TMT 2 joint cannot be clarified sufficiently using sonography.

Stress fractures are only visible if the cortex is also affected. In the case of older fractures callus activity with a bulge thickening of the bone line can be seen first on the ultrasound image and only later on an X-ray image (Fig. 18.8a, b).

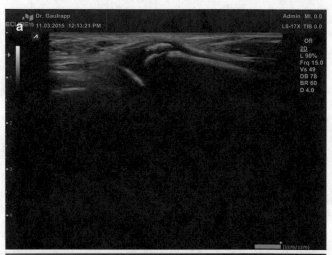

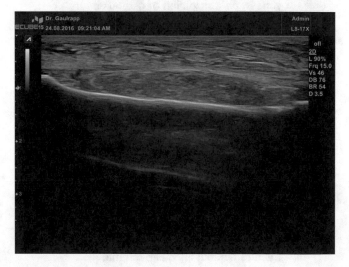

Fig. 18.1 (a, b) Normal apophysis nucleus in a 12-year-old child in a sonogram and in an X-ray image

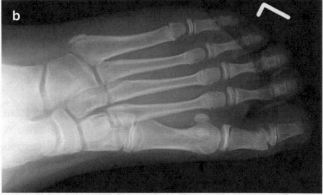

Fig. 18.2 Echo-rich periosteal hematoma over the MT 2, bone intact

18.5.5 Diagnosis

If there is sonographic evidence of an osseous injury, this must be confirmed in a two plane X-ray image. Questionable stress lesions that do not show any sonographically visible lesion of the cortex and can be an indication for magnetic resonance imaging. Sonography of fractures on the foot does not currently replace X-ray diagnostics.

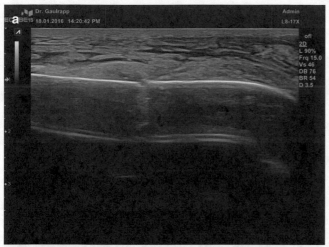

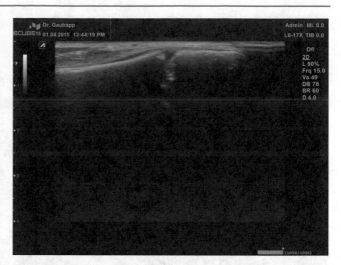

Fig. 18.5 Salter/Harris fracture 1 in a child with a periostal hematoma

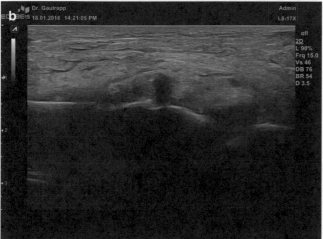

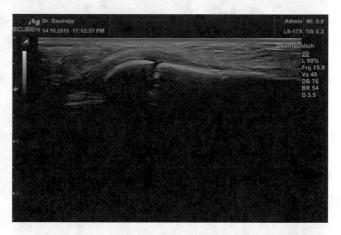

Fig. 18.3 (**a**) Outer ankle fracture in the fibular LS with a clear gap and echo-rich periosteal hematoma. (**b**) Anterior LS to (**a**) shows the cortical interruption with a periostal hematoma

Fig. 18.6 Cross fracture of the base of the metatarsal 5. The Peroneus brevis tendon runs unharmed over the fracture gap

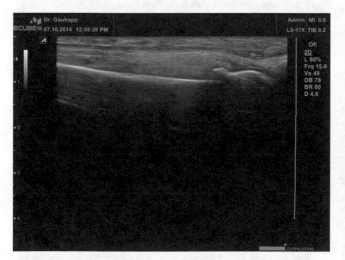

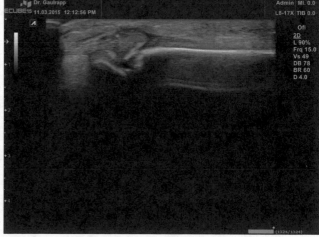

Fig. 18.4 Subcapital fracture at metatarsal 2 with clearly visible kink formation

Fig. 18.7 Avulsion fracture in a 12-year-old child (see Fig. 18.1) with a tear in the Peronäus brevis tendon

18.5.6 Therapy and Controls

If there are bony injuries, a final X-ray check is carried out depending on the age of the patient. Sonographic check-ups are not necessary.

18.6 Pitfalls and Red Flags

If bony injuries are suspected even though there was no adequate trauma, sonography is a good screening method to

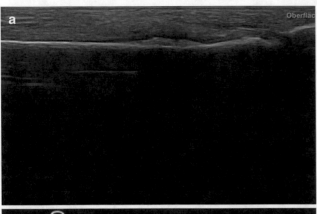

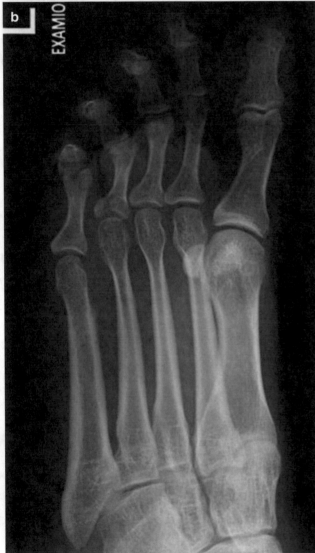

Complex traumas, especially with soft tissue and skin injuries, pose particular challenges for clinical and imaging diagnostics. Sonography is of far less importance here.

Sonography proves to be helpful for the differential diagnosis of whether adjacent tarsal joints or basic toe joints are injured when assessing a hemarthrosis or torn ligaments, especially since sonography allows the detection of joint instabilities.

Isolated internal bone lesions cannot be assessed sonographically or radiologically. Usually, magnetic resonance tomography can help here. Systemic diseases that affect the calcification of the bone or that are associated with multiple bone changes make imaging diagnostics difficult.

If despite an inconspicuous primary ultrasound examination symptoms persist after 7 days, a sonographic check-up or a further radiological examination should be carried out.

Further Reading

1. Atilla OD, Yesilaras M, Kilic TY, Tur FC, Reisoglu A, Sever M, Aksay E. The accuracy of bedside ultrasonography as a diagnostic tool for fractures in the ankle and foot. Acad Emerg Med. 2014;21:1058–61.
2. Battaglia PJ, Kaeser MA, Kettner NW. Diagnosis and serial sonography of a proximal fifth metatarsal stress fracture. J Chiropr Med. 2013;12(3):196–200.
3. Bianchi S, Luong DH. Stress fractures of the calcaneus diagnosed by sonography: report of 8 cases. J Ultrasound Med. 2017;37:521. https://doi.org/10.1002/jum.14276. [Epub ahead of print].
4. Canagasabey MD, Callaghan MJ, Carley S. The sonographic Ottawa foot and ankle rules study (the SOFAR study). Emerg Med J. 2011;28(10):838–40.
5. Ekinci S, Polat O, Günalp M, Demirkan A, Koca A. The accuracy of ultrasound evaluation in foot and ankle trauma. Am J Emerg Med. 2013;31(11):1551–5.
6. Hatch RL, Alsobrook JA, Clugston JR. Diagnosis and management of metatarsal fractures. Am Acad Fam Phys. 2007;76(6):817–26.
7. Hedelin H, Goksör LÅ, Karlsson J, Stjernström S. Ultrasound-assisted triage of ankle trauma can decrease the need for radiographic imaging. Am J Emerg Med. 2013;31(12):1686–9.
8. Hofsli M, Torfing T, Al-Aubaidi Z. The proportion of distal fibula Salter-Harris type I epiphyseal fracture in the paediatric population with acute ankle injury: a prospective MRI study. J Pediatr Orthop B. 2016;25(2):126–32.
9. Hübner U, Schlicht W, Outzen S, Barthel M, Halsband H. Ultrasound in the diagnosis of fractures in children. J Bone Joint Surg Br. 2000;82(8):1170–3.
10. Kozaci N, Ay MO, Avci M, Beydilli I, Turhan S, Donertas E, Ararat E. The comparison of radiography and point-of-care ultrasonography in the diagnosis and management of metatarsal fractures. Injury. 2017;48(2):542–7.
11. Oh MJ, Park KT, Youn KM, Joo JC, Park SJ. Color Doppler sonography accompanied by dynamic scanning for the diagnosis of ankle and foot fractures. J Ultrasound Med. 2018;37(6):1555–64.
12. Robertson NB, Roocroft JH, Edmonds EW. Childhood metatarsal shaft fractures: treatment outcomes and relative indications for surgical intervention. J Child Orthop. 2012;6:125–9.
13. Tollefson B, Nichols J, Fromang S, Summers RL. Validation of the sonographic Ottawa foot and ankle rules (SOFAR) study in a large urban trauma center. J Miss State Med Assoc. 2016;57(2):35–8.
14. Yesilaras M, Aksay E, Atilla OD, Sever M, Kalenderer O. The accuracy of bedside ultrasonography as a diagnostic tool for the fifth metatarsal fractures. Am J Emerg Med. 2014;32(2):171–4.

Fig. 18.8 (**a**) Advanced stress fracture distal to metatarsal 5 with an echogenic cortical reaction and subperiostal edema. (**b**) X-ray image for (**a**)

differentiate soft tissue injuries, superficial bony injuries, and joint injuries close to the bone. Previous injuries should also make the examiner aware of whether an extended diagnostic clarification, including imaging, could be necessary.

Screening for Lower Extremity Fractures

19

Kolja Eckert

19.1   Synopsis

1.1 Indication: sonographic primary evaluation for traumatically caused painful limping in toddlers; toddler fracture suspected.

1.2 Rationale of application: X-ray-free diagnosis and therapy for injuries to the lower extremity in childhood. Narrowing down the region of interest.

1.3 Contraindications: open fractures, V.a. accompanying vascular/nerve injuries, clearly visible malposition, safe surgical indication.

1.4 Age of the patient: 0–8 years.

1.5 Examination: medical history, clinical examination, ultrasound: sonographic representation of the hip joint (ventral longitudinal section) and the femur and tibia from at least three projections.

1.6 Indications for additional X-ray diagnostics:
– sonographic fracture detection with dislocation.
– clinical suspicion of a fracture of the foot skeleton.
– persistent pain, even if no fracture was found sonographically.
– uncertainty in the assessment.
– refractures.

1.7 Pitfalls:
– benign or malignant bone tumors.
– osteomyelitis, septic arthritis.
– child abuse.
– bone metabolism disorders (e.g., osteogenesis imperfecta).
– children's rheumatological diseases.
– pediatric orthopedic diseases: M. Perthes (ages 5–9), epiphysolysis capitis femoris (ages 10–14), Osgood-Schlatter (ages 9–14), aseptic bone necrosis.

1.8 Red flags:
– painless limping.
– severe pain/immobility even without fracture detection.
– fracture without adequate trauma.
– pre-traumatic complaints at the appropriate location.
– increasing complaints under therapy.

19.2   Introduction

Painful limping in toddlers (<5 years) is a common reason for introducing pediatric emergency consultations. This summarizes the consequences of injuries, which mostly result from low-energy trauma and for which the clinical symptoms can be very discreet.

A typical consequence of an injury is the so-called toddler fracture. Toddler fractures typically occur in children between the ages of 9 months and 3 years of age, more rarely in children up to the age of 8. The injury mechanism is usually characterized by a torsion event, so that undisplaced spiral fractures occur in the area of the distal two-thirds of the tibia in 95% of the cases. The femur can also be affected, but much less frequently.

Another typical consequence of injuries is metaphyseal torus fractures of the distal femur and the proximal or distal tibia. These are compression fractures, which can also occur after jumping from a low height. These are also mostly undislocated fractures.

Both types of injury can also pose a diagnostic challenge for the experienced examiner. If directly observed by the parents, these accidents are mostly described as seemingly banal twisting or twisting trauma. Owing to a frequently unclear

K. Eckert (✉)
Marienhospital Gelsenkirchen, Klinik für Kinderchirurgie,
Gelsenkirchen, Germany
e-mail: K.Eckert@marienhospital.eu

© Springer Nature Switzerland AG 2021
O. Ackermann (ed.), *Fracture Sonography*, https://doi.org/10.1007/978-3-030-63839-9_19

medical history and the lack of typical clinical signs of fracture such as swelling, hematoma, or malposition, an actual underlying fracture, even on the part of the doctor, can be underestimated.

After the initial pain event, the child appears to calm down quickly, an analgesic may also help. But the child does not become completely symptom-free. Most of the time, in the otherwise unaffected child, a painful limp or a persistent refusal to walk is noticeable, which ultimately leads to a medical presentation even after a few days.

The clinical assessment is sometimes made difficult by the fact that small children often cannot provide precise information about the location of the pain or that the child does not allow an exact examination due to anxiety. Nevertheless, careful and subtle palpation at the predilection sites for a suspected fracture is always a prerequisite for the most accurate imaging possible. For radiological reasons, X-rays of the entire leg and hip should be avoided as far as possible, especially since an initially unremarkable X-ray image cannot always rule out a fracture that is actually present, especially in toddler fractures. It is not uncommon for such a fracture to be confirmed as a discrete periosteal callus reaction in the X-ray control after 10–14 days if the symptoms persist.

If there is no traumatic cause in the classic case, coxitis fugax is another important differential diagnosis for painful limping. Coxitis fugax usually occurs parainfectious and leads to a painful, gentle posture of the affected leg in a slight abduction, flexion, and external rotation position. The cause is a serious hip joint effusion, which leads to painful joint capsule tension with sometimes complete refusal to walk. Protection and analgesic-anti-inflammatory therapy is the therapy of choice.

With coxitis fugax, ultrasound imaging is the first choice. In the case of systemic signs of infection, however, further clarification is necessary in order to reliably rule out septic arthritis.

Bone lesions in childhood always show an involvement of the bone surface (bulging, cortical interruption, etc.), which can be displayed very sensitively using sonography. Ultrasound thus offers a sensible alternative to a primary evaluation in the event of suspected fracture of the lower extremity, thus enabling an X-ray-free diagnosis or at least a targeted limitation of the X-ray examination.

19.3   Indication

Basically, the ultrasound can be used for primary evaluation as a screening in every toddler who is presented with painful limps. With the sound probe, the entire limb is scanned from the hip joint to the knee to the distal lower leg. If there is a sonographic fracture detection or if there is diagnostic uncertainty, an additional X-ray examination can be arranged. In the case of sonographic fracture exclusion, however, an X-ray examination can be dispensed with for the time being.

19.4   Indications for X-ray Diagnostics

Clinical experience shows that the typical bead and toddler fractures of the femur or tibia heal easily and without consequences under conservative therapy (immobilization in the cast association). Basically, the sole ultrasound is also suitable for therapy control in these cases with reliable fracture diagnosis. A confirmatory X-ray examination does not result in any diagnostic added value. However, there are still insufficient comparative studies available. For this reason, a targeted X-ray examination of the corresponding bone section is to be discussed at present with sonographic fracture detection. An additional X-ray imaging should therefore only be dispensed with after extensive clarification and with the consent of the parents.

Sonography is particularly suitable for the detection of fractures in the area of long bones. With the short (tubular) bones of the foot skeleton, however, the diagnostic significance of ultrasound clearly decreases. In the case of an accident mechanism similar to that of the bead fractures, if a femoral or lower leg fracture is clinically and sonographically excluded and the gait is obviously refused, metatarsal lesions must be considered as the next probable cause. Sonographic metatarsal imaging can be achieved under suitable examination conditions, but documentation of the findings in a restless child can be difficult, so that if there is clinical suspicion and after fracture exclusion of the femur and tibia, a targeted X-ray examination of the foot should be considered.

If symptoms persist or even increase during therapy, an X-ray examination should be carried out. If in doubt, new sonography will show no result other than the primary examination, and therefore, appears to be unnecessary.

19.5   Examination

By carefully palpating the affected limb, an attempt is first made to clinically limit the location of the fracture on the affected limb. Particular attention should be paid to the typical cortical tapping and pressure pain, to discrete swellings, and also subtle hematomas at the known predilection sites. This is followed directly by the sonographic examination, which is preferably carried out from proximal, starting above the hip joint, to distal.

Fig. 19.1 Screening-SAFE. (©Ackermann and Eckert 2015; Courtesy of off label media)

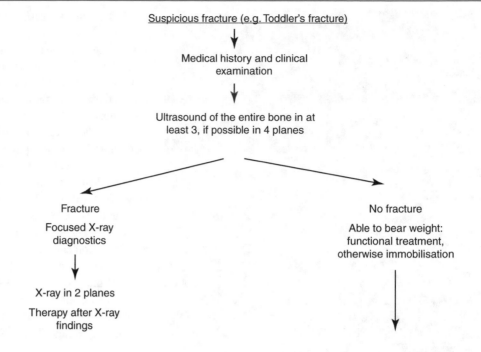

<u>Suspicious fracture (e.g. Toddler's fracture)</u>

↓

Medical history and clinical examination

↓

Ultrasound of the entire bone in at least 3, if possible in 4 planes

Fracture

Focused X-ray diagnostics

↓

X-ray in 2 planes

Therapy after X-ray findings

No fracture

Able to bear weight: functional treatment, otherwise immobilisation

↓

Clinical follow-up after 5 days, in case of persistent complaints X-ray control

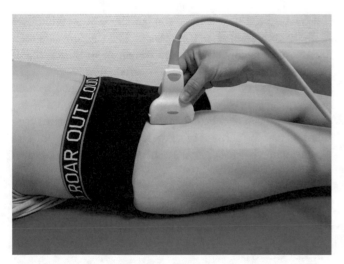

Fig. 19.2 Patient positioning for ventral hip ultrasound. (©Ackermann and Eckert 2015; Courtesy of off label media)

19.5.1 Positioning

For the ventral hip ultrasound to detect or exclude a hip joint effusion, the patient must be placed on the back (Fig. 19.1). Otherwise, there are no requirements for the positioning of children. After a sonographic examination of a possible hip effusion, the little patient can sit or lie on the examination couch as he likes, next to or on the lap of the parents (Fig. 19.2).

When the child is sitting or lying down, the respective dorsal planes cannot be adjusted without additional repositioning measures or manipulations on the affected limb.

19.5.2 Views

A hip joint effusion is detected or excluded using a ventral longitudinal view over the hip joint (Fig. 19.1). For the femur, tibia, and fibula, it is important to display these from at least three, if possible from four projections (ventral, lateral, dorsal, and medial). The probe guidance from proximal to distal enables a dynamic and almost complete (multiplanar) assessment of the respective cortex. For documentation purposes, the findings must be recorded in all projections. This corresponds to the anteroposterior and lateral levels of a standard X-ray examination.

Starting at the hip joint, the femur is first examined from proximal to distal using the sonic probe. The child can sit down again if the examination conditions are easier. The most accessible are the ventral, lateral (e.g., Fig. 19.3), and medial projections. In addition to the ventral view of the metaphyseal cortex, the suprapatellar longitudinal section also enables a possible knee joint effusion to be assessed (Fig. 19.4). On the knee joint, the femoral and tibial metaphyses can be easily adjusted from all four directions. The tibial shaft can then be moved from the ventromedial and the distal tibial metaphysis and the fibula can be shown from the ventral, lateral, and dorsal. Toddler fractures and metaphyseal bead fractures can thus be detected or excluded very well at their predilection sites. However, the course of the examination is left to the current examination situation and the examiner according to the individual preference.

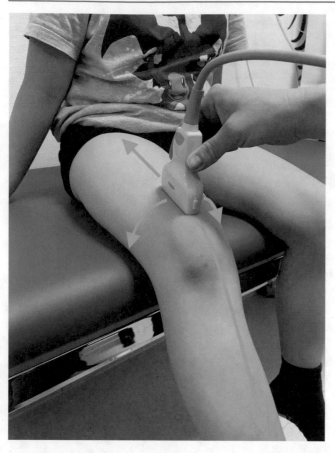

Fig. 19.3 Patient positioning for sonographic examination of the lower extremity. (©Ackermann and Eckert 2015; Courtesy of off label media)

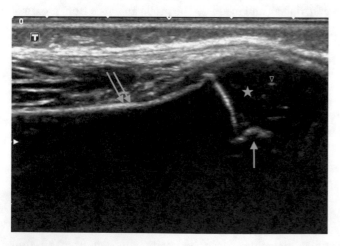

Fig. 19.4 Lateral longitudinal section over the distal femoral metaphysis, boy 2 years old; the uninjured cortex (double arrow) is curved homogeneously, the epiphyseal cartilage (asterisk) appears almost anechoic; small anechoic reflexes (arrowhead) correspond to cartilage cell islands; the epiphyseal core (arrow) shows a physiologically irregular surface on the side facing the transducer. (©Ackermann and Eckert 2015; Courtesy of off label media)

19.5.3 Assessment

A hip joint effusion can be assessed via the proximal femoral metaphysis of the femoral neck. The joint capsule normally runs parallel to the femoral cortex (Fig. 19.5a). With coxitis fugax, there is anechoic effusion in the inferior recess of the joint capsule and lifts it convexly to the ventricle (Fig. 19.5b). However, there are no reliable sonographic criteria for a safe differentiation from septic arthritis.

Child fractures always result in a sonographically representable lesion of the bone surface. In this way, kink and bulge fractures can be distinguished (Figs. 19.6, 19.7a, b, 19.8, and 19.9). But also cortical interruptions (Figs. 19.7c, 19.10, 19.11, 19.12) with or without a noticeable offset or an axis deviation can be recognized.

The typical torus and toddler fractures show no dislocation. In these cases, there is no need to measure the axis deviation because an additional measurement of the axis deviation is unnecessary if there is apparently no dislocation in the X-ray image (Figs. 19.13, 19.14, 19.15, and 19.16).

19.5.4 Diagnosis and Therapy

If a fracture can be excluded sonographically, an additional X-ray examination is not necessary. The therapy is symptomatic using analgesia, reduced weight-bearing, and possibly also immobilization in the cast association.

In the case of sonographic diagnosis of an undisplaced metaphyseal torus- or toddler fracture, an additional X-ray examination can also be dispensed with after extensive consultation and the consent of the parents. The therapy follows the current pediatric surgical standard and usually consists of cast immobilization for about 2–4 weeks.

X-ray examination is mandatory for shaft fractures with misalignment or axial deviation that are proven by ultrasound.

19.5.5 Controls

Even after initial sonographic exclusion of fractures, persistent or even progressive complaints should be followed by a targeted X-ray check after 7 days at the latest.

If the torus- or toddler fracture is proven, the cast is immobilized for about 2–4 weeks. After the application of the cast, there is only a clinical check. In the absence of local callus pressure or palpating pain, the therapy is stopped, and if the symptoms persist, immobilization is prolonged. Imaging position or consolidation checks during the course, both sonographically and radiologically, are not necessary, since the duration of the immobilization depends on the clinical symptoms.

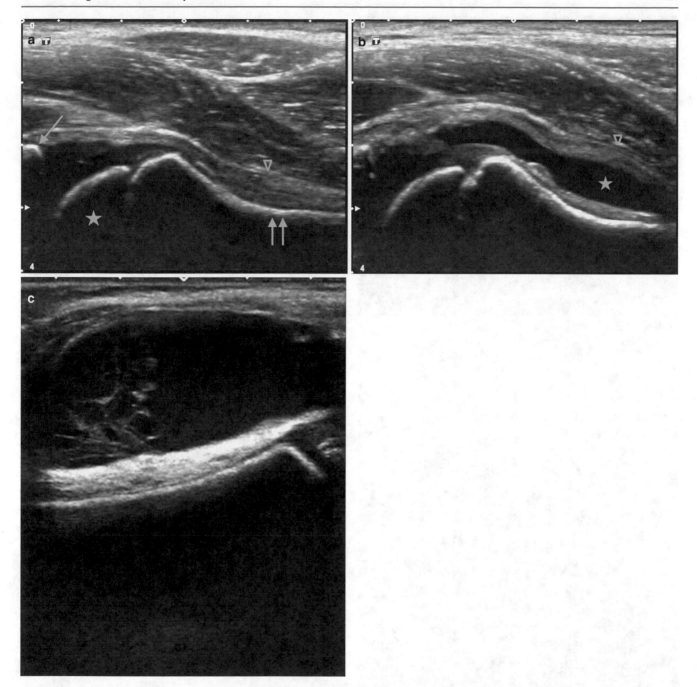

Fig. 19.5 Hip comparison effusion (coxitis fugax) in side comparison. (**a**) Left hip joint without effusion, acetabulum (arrow), epiphysis (asterisk), the joint capsule (arrow head) runs parallel to the cortex (double arrow), without effusion, the synovial lies against each other. (**b**) Right hip joint with anechoic effusion (asterisk) in the inferior recess, the ventral hip joint capsule (arrow head) lifts convexly towards the ventral. (**c**) Knee effusion, boy 11 years old; suprapatellar longitudinal section over the ventral femoral metaphysis; the superior recess is biconvex, the effusion is inhomogeneously echo-rich and is, therefore, an urgent indication of damage to the knee. (©Ackermann and Eckert 2015; Courtesy of off label media)

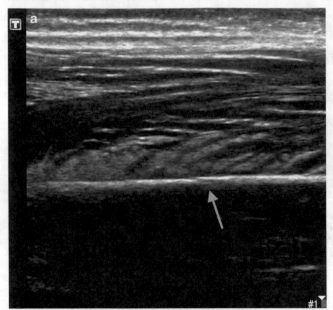

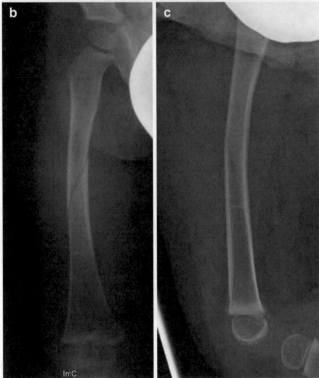

Fig. 19.6 Toddler fracture of the femoral shaft, boy 5 years old; ultrasound (**a**) ventral US longitudinal section over the middle third of the femoral shaft, discreet but still easily visible cortical disruption (arrow), and (**b** and **c**) corresponding X-ray image. (©Ackermann and Eckert 2015; Courtesy of off label media)

In the case of displaced, possibly osteosynthetically treated shaft fractures, clinical, and radiological controls are carried out in accordance with the standard for traumatology in children.

19.6   Pitfalls and Red Flags

An accurate medical history and subtle clinical examination determine the indication for the most suitable imaging, and thus, a correct diagnosis and adequate therapy. However, the correct diagnosis does not primarily depend on the selected imaging, but rather on the interpretation of the findings in conjunction with the anamnestic and clinical findings.

For example, toddler fractures in particular can be difficult to detect on the X-ray. Therefore, it is basically the case that injuries with a suspected fracture should be treated appropriately even without fracture correlate.

Proper handling of suspected child abuse is always an interdisciplinary challenge and ultrasound can be used to search for fresh fractures. Nevertheless, the detection of older, already consolidated fractures is reserved for X-ray diagnostics.

In the case of medical history and clinical examination, attention must be paid to appropriate warning signals, which may also indicate a nontraumatic cause for the limping in order to select the appropriate imaging method.

Painful limping without adequate trauma can result in pediatric orthopedic diseases (e.g., Perthes' disease, epiphyseolysis capitis femoris, Osgood-Schlatter's disease aseptic bone necrosis), rheumatological or infectious diseases (e.g., osteomyelitis), and painless gentle limping. The primary ultrasound examination can also provide valuable information in these cases. However, in the event of anamnestic, clinical, and diagnostic uncertainty, it should be consistently supplemented by further and suitable imaging (e.g., X-ray, CT, MRI).

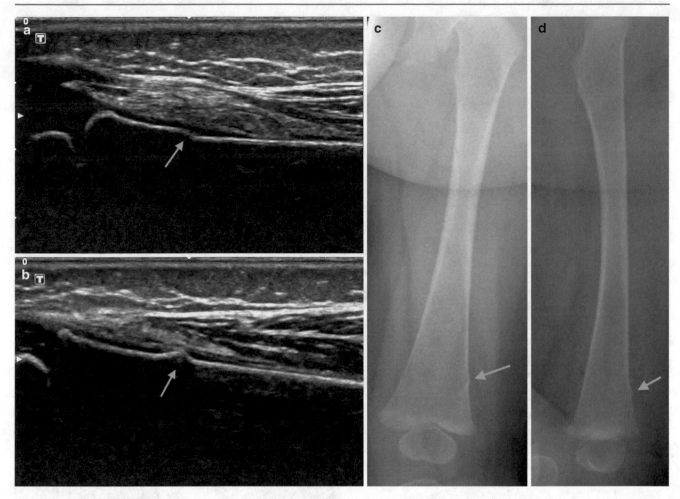

Fig. 19.7 Metaphyseal bulge fracture of the distal femur (arrow), boy 6 years old; ultrasound (**a**) ventral longitudinal section, (**b**) medial longitudinal section, and (**c** and **d**) corresponding X-ray image. (©Ackermann and Eckert 2015; Courtesy of off label media)

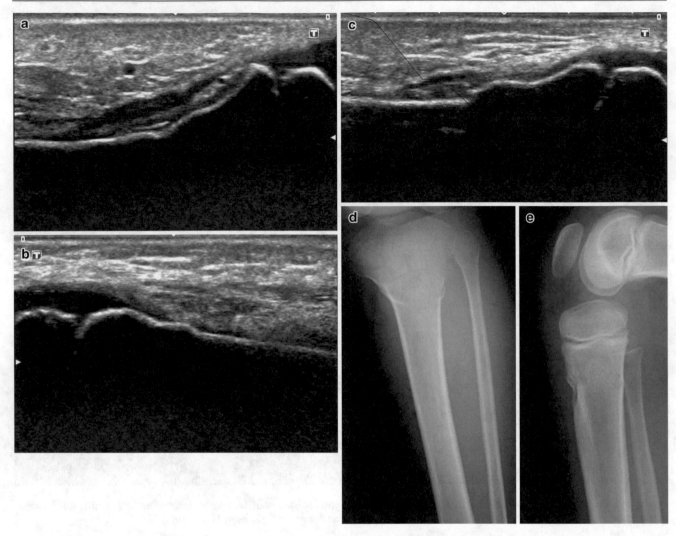

Fig. 19.8 Proximal tibia bulge fracture (arrow), girl 8 years old; ultrasound (**a**) medial longitudinal section, (**b**) lateral longitudinal section, (**c**) ventral longitudinal section, and (**d** and **e**) corresponding X-ray image. (©Ackermann and Eckert 2015; Courtesy of off label media)

Fig. 19.9 Left tibia toddler fracture (arrow), boy 3 years old. (**a**) ultrasound, ventromedial longitudinal section over the distal third of the tibia, clearly visible cortical interruption without significant misalignment or kinking and (**b**) corresponding X-ray image. (©Ackermann and Eckert 2015; Courtesy of off label media)

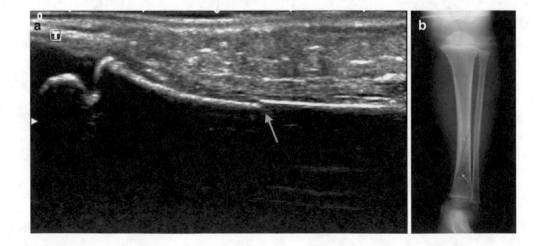

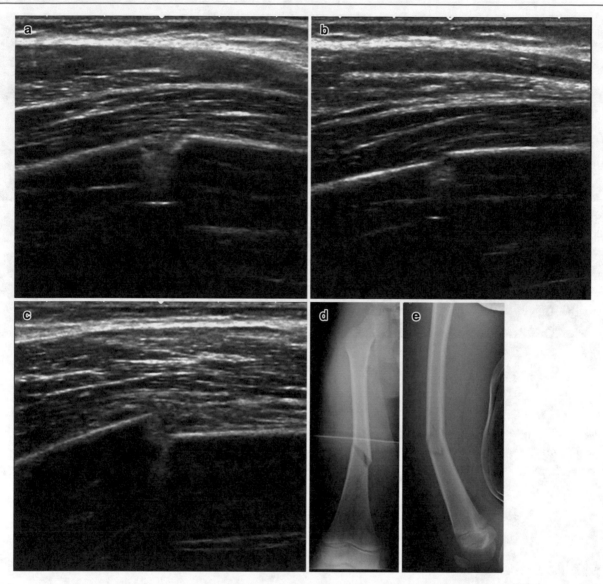

Fig. 19.10 Femoral shaft fracture, girl 7 years old; Ultrasonic longitudinal sections over the middle third of the femur (**a**) from the ventral, (**b**) from the lateral, (**c**) from the medial, an interruption of the cortex and kinking are clearly visible, and (**d** and **e**) corresponding X-ray image. (©Ackermann and Eckert 2015; Courtesy of off label media)

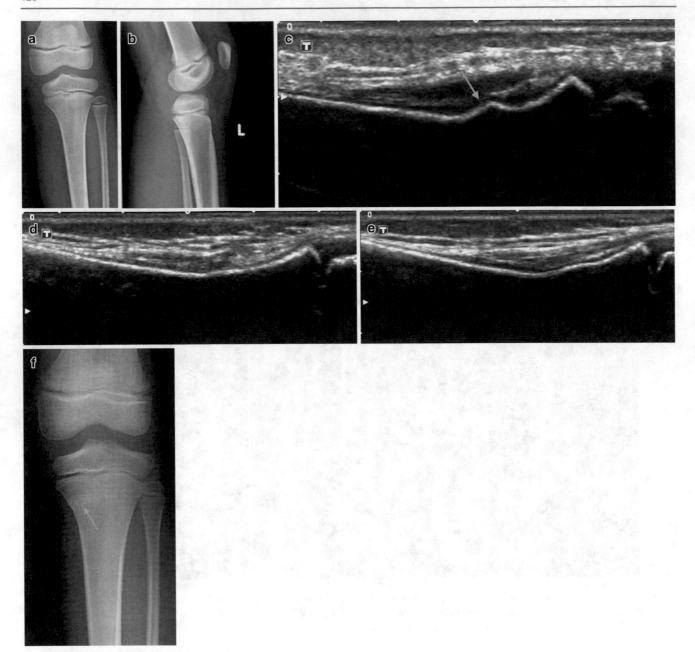

Fig. 19.11 Proximal tibia bead fractures, girl 7 years old, no memorable trauma, but extensive trampoline jumping the day before, now pain in the area of the left knee. (**a** and **b**) X-ray image at first presentation, no visible signs of fracture, (**c**) ventromedial ultrasound longitudinal section over the proximal tibia, clearly visible bulging (arrow), (**d**) for comparison ventromedial ultrasound longitudinal section over the proximal tibia contralateral, homogeneously curved cortex without visible cortical lesion; 18 days later, (**e**) Longitudinal ventromedial ultrasound cut over the proximal tibia, markedly receding bulging, and (**f**) corresponding X-ray image: a discrete sclerotic zone (arrow) shows on the medial cortex as a sign of a fracture that has taken place. (©Ackermann and Eckert 2015; Courtesy of off label media)

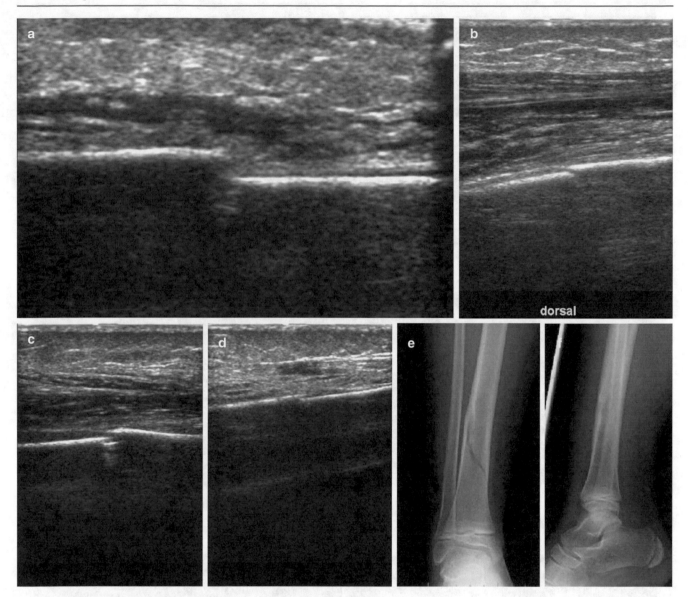

Fig. 19.12 Slightly dislocated tibia shaft fracture. Ultrasound (**a**) ventral, (**b**) dorsal, (**c**) lateral, (**d**) medial, clearly visible cortical interruption with discrete misalignment and kinking, and (**e** and **f**) corresponding X-ray image. (©Ackermann and Eckert 2015; Courtesy of off label media)

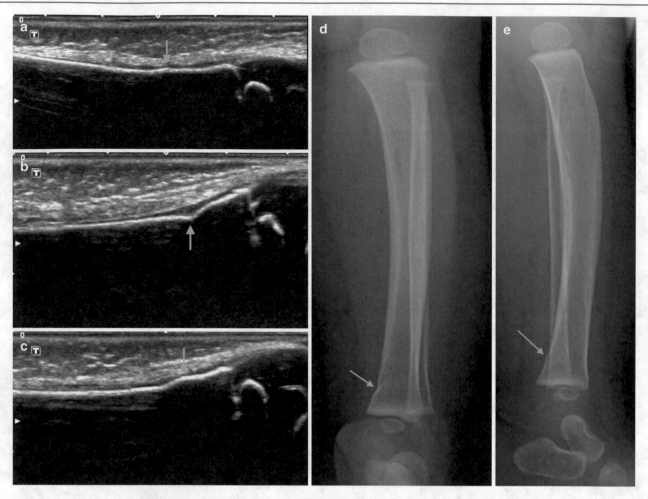

Fig. 19.13 (**a** and **b**) Distal tibia bead fracture (arrow), boy 2 years old; ultrasound: (**a**) from ventral, (**b**) from medial, (**c**) from lateral, and (**d** and **e**) corresponding X-ray image. (©Ackermann and Eckert 2015; Courtesy of off label media)

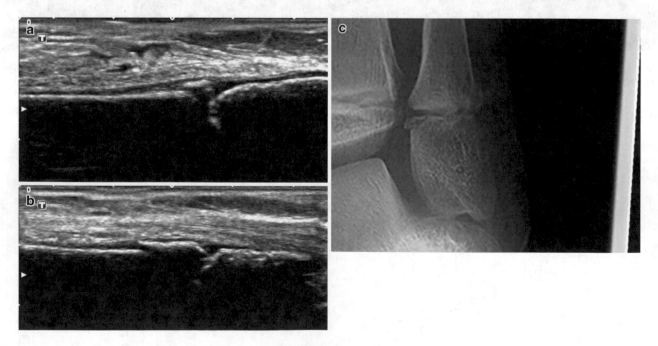

Fig. 19.14 Distal fibular epiphyseal fracture (arrow) type Aitken-1, boy 9 years old. (**a**) ultrasound: lateral projection, (**b**) dorsal projection, and (**c**) corresponding X-ray image. (©Ackermann and Eckert 2015; Courtesy of off label media)

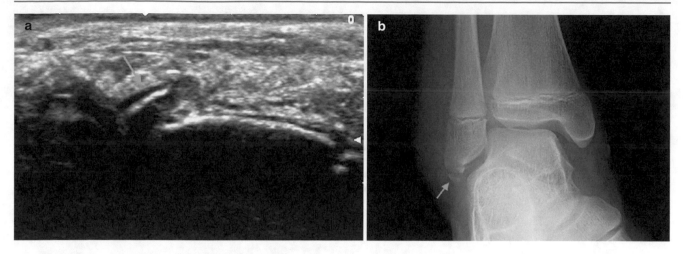

Fig. 19.15 Flake fracture (arrow) of the distal fibular epiphysis, boy 13 years old. (**a**) ultrasound: lateral projection and (**b**) corresponding X-ray image. (©Ackermann and Eckert 2015; Courtesy of off label media)

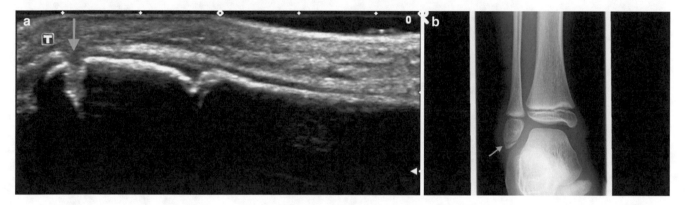

Fig. 19.16 A bony tear of the distal fibula (arrow), girl 7 years old. (**a**) Ultrasound: lateral projection and (**b**) corresponding X-ray image. (©Ackermann and Eckert 2015; Courtesy of off label media)

Further Reading

1. Abi KS, Haddad-Zebouni S, Roukoz S, et al. Ultrasound as an adjunct to radiography in minor musculoskeletal pediatric trauma. J Med Liban. 2011;59(2):70–4.
2. Barata I, Spencer R, Suppiah A, et al. Emergency ultrasound in the detection of pediatric long-bone fractures. Pediatr Emerg Care. 2012;28:1154–7.
3. Beltrame V, Stramarea R, Rebellatoa N, et al. Sonographic evaluation of bone fractures: a reliable alternative in clinical practice? Clin Imaging. 2012;36:203–8.
4. Bienvenu-Perrard M, de Suremain N, Wicart PJ, et al. Benefit of hip ultrasound in management of the limping child. Radiol. 2007;88(3 Pt 1):377–83.
5. Deanehan J, Gallagher R, Vieira R, et al. Bedside hip ultrasonography in the pediatric emergency department: a tool to guide management in patients presenting with limp. Pediatr Emerg Care. 2014;30(4):285–7.
6. Gleeson AP, Stuart MJ, Wilson B, et al. Ultrasound assessment and conservative management of inversion injuries of the ankle in children: plaster of Paris versus Tubigrip. J Bone Joint Surg Br. 1996;78(3):484–7.
7. Graif M, Stahl-Kent V, Ben-Ami T, et al. Sonographic detection of occult bone fractures. Pediatr Radiol. 1988;18(5):383–5.
8. Hübner U, Schlicht W, Outzen S, et al. Ultrasound in the diagnosis of fractures in children. J Bone Joint Surg Br. 2000;82(8):1170–3.
9. Jones S, Colaco K, Fischer J, et al. Accuracy of point-of-care ultrasonography for pediatric ankle sprain injuries. Pediatr Emerg Care. 2018;34(12):842–7.
10. Kozacia N, Ayb MO, Avcia M, et al. The comparison of radiography and point-of-care ultrasonography in the diagnosis and management of metatarsal fractures. Injury. 2017;48:542–7.
11. Lewis D, Logan P. Sonographic diagnosis of toddler's fracture in the emergency department. J Clin Ultrasound. 2006;34:190–4.
12. Maeda M, Maeda N, Takaoka T. Sonographic findings of chondral avulsion fractures of the lateral ankle ligaments in children. J Ultrasound Med. 2017;36:421–32.
13. Markowitz RI, Hubbard AM, Harty MP, et al. Sonography of the knee in normal and abused infants. Pediatr Radiol. 1993;23(4):264–7.
14. Moritz JD, Berthold LD, Soenksen SF, et al. Ultrasound in diagnosis of fractures in children: unnecessary harassment or useful addition to X-ray? Ultraschall Med. 2008;29:267–74.

15. Moritz JD, Hoffmann B, Meuser SH, et al. Is ultrasound equal to X-ray in pediatric fracture diagnosis? Fortschr Röntgenstr. 2010;182:706–14.

16. Patel DD, Blumberg SM, Crain EF. The utility of bedside ultrasonography in identifying fractures and guiding fracture reduction in children. Pediatr Emerg Care. 2009;25:221–5.

17. Rathfelder FJ, Paar O. Ultrasound as an alternative diagnostic measure for fractures during the growth phase. Unfallchirurg. 1995;98:645–9.

18. Rathfelder FJ, Paar O. Possibilities for using sonography as a diagnostic procedure in fractures during the growth period. Unfallchirurg. 1995;98:645–9.

19. Simanovsky N, Lamdan R, Hiller N, et al. Sonographic detection of radiographically occult fractures in pediatric ankle and wrist injuries. J Pediatr Orthop. 2005;29(2):142–5.

20. Simanovsky N, Hiller N, Leibner E, et al. Sonographic detection of radiographically occult fractures in paediatric ankle injuries. Pediatr Radiol. 2005;35:1062–5.

21. Steiner GM, Sprigg A. The value of ultrasound in the assessment of bone. Br J Radiol. 1992 Jul;65(775):589–93.

22. Warkentine F, Horowitz R, Pierce MC. The use of ultrasound to detect occult or unsuspected fractures in child abuse. Pediatr Emerg Care. 2014;30(1):43–6.

23. Wang CL, Shieh JY, Wang TG, et al. Sonographic detection of occult fractures in the foot and ankle. J Clin Ultrasound. 1999;27(8):421–5.

24. Weinberg ER, Tunik MG, Tsung JW. Accuracy of clinician-performed point-of-care ultrasound for the diagnosis of fractures in children and young adults. Injury. 2010;41:862–8.

Part III

General Indications

Ole Ackermann

20.1 Synopsis

1.1 Rationale of application: exclusion of an axis deviation from the shaft and metaphyseal fractures during treatment.

1.2 Evidence level: IV.

1.3 Indications: stable, conservatively treated, and osteosynthetically treated fractures of the shaft and metaphysis.

1.4 Contraindications: joint fractures, loosening of material, closed plaster.

1.5 Age of the patient: any age.

1.6 Examination: representation of at least three, if possible four levels.

1.7 Indications for additional X-ray diagnostics:
   – evidence of an axis deviation.
   – planned surgery.
   – uncertainty in the assessment.
   – question about the material situation/material breakage.
   – problem infection/loosening.

1.8 Pitfalls:
   – short image sections with long bones.
   – overlay by osteosynthesis material.

1.9 Red flags:
   – increasing complaints under therapy.
   – infection sign.

1.10 Algorithm: Follow-up SAFE.

20.2 Introduction

Sonographic position checks have been published time and again, especially in the reduction control of distal radius fractures. Although there are no large, directly comparative studies, the use of this technique seems safe and sufficient against the background of experience with other indications (Fig. 20.1).

Fracture sonography shows bone surfaces of all limb bones and allows sufficient axis determination. It is, therefore, also useful to use it for bone fractures that have already been diagnosed and even treated with osteosynthesis. The question here is the pure axis determination, that is, the exclusion of an increasing axis deviation in the course of therapy. This is particularly important for conservatively treated fractures and special fracture entities (e.g., MFK 5 base fracture).

This type of diagnostics requires a lot of experience in dealing with these lesions in order to correctly interpret red flags to ensure safe treatment.

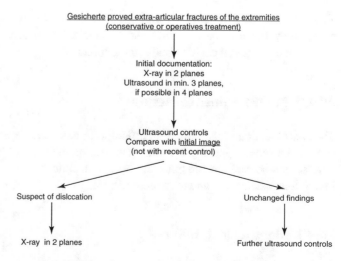

Fig. 20.1 Follow-up SAFE. (©Ole Ackermann 2020. All rights reserved)

O. Ackermann (✉)
Department of Orthopedic Surgery, Ruhr-University Bochum, Bochum, Germany

© Springer Nature Switzerland AG 2021
O. Ackermann (ed.), *Fracture Sonography*, https://doi.org/10.1007/978-3-030-63839-9_20

20.3 Indication Including Patient Age

All bone fractures of the extremities in the shaft or metaphyseal area are suitable for sonographic control, regardless of the age of the patient. Sufficient imaging must have taken place, ideally with an X-ray and sonographic examination on day 0.

Sonography only answers the question of dislocation and an axis deviation. Sufficient statements regarding the osteosynthesis material or the occurrence of infections cannot be made.

Typical indications are:

- extremity fractures in children; these are often treated conservatively and have very good healing potential.
- MFK 5 base fracture in adults; here the indication for surgery is often made in the course when the fragment dislocates; the diagnosis is complicated by the fact that it is often difficult radiologically to repeat the settings of the comparison picture exactly; sonography always represents the maximum axis deviation and is very suitable for monitoring the course.
- radial head fractures; reproducing the setting of a comparative picture is also problematic here. The radius head can be represented sonographically and rotated dynamically under the transducer so that sufficient statements can be made here (Figs. 20.2, 20.3, and 20.4).
- simple shaft fractures of the extremities in adults; axis determination is also essential here. This can be assessed well sonographically.

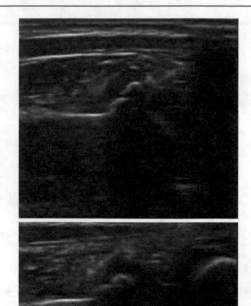

Fig. 20.2 and 20.3 Left radial head fracture in longitudinal sonographic section; right inside rotation. (©Ackermann and Eckert 2015; Courtesy of off label media)

20.4 Contraindications and Indications for X-ray Diagnostics

20.4.1 Articular Fractures

The assessment of intra-articular findings is not possible with sonography. In particular, no reliable statements can be made regarding the material position and fragment reduction.

20.4.2 Multi-fragment Fractures

The exact location of individual superficial fragments can be shown in a sonographically complex manner, but the procedure is time-consuming and not reliably reproducible. X-ray imaging is faster, safer, and more comparable.

20.4.3 Material Instability

Osteosynthesis material is sonographically shadowing and sound-canceling. Intraosseous parts cannot be displayed so

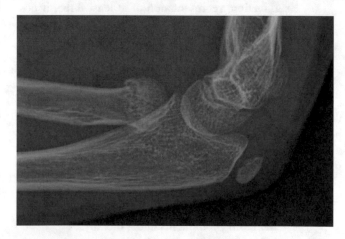

Fig. 20.4 Radius head fracture from Figs. 20.2 and 20.3 in the side X-ray image. (©Ackermann and Eckert 2015; Courtesy of off label media)

that the assessment of metal implants is a domain of X-ray imaging.

20.4.4 Infection Situation

In the infection situation, there is always the question of bone involvement, which cannot be adequately answered by sonography.

20.4.5 Consolidation Controls

The superficial callus formation can be visualized sono-graphically, but the filling of fracture gaps cannot. Ultrasound technology is, therefore, not suitable for sufficient consolidation control.

20.4.6 Examination

Diagnostics and therapy follow the follow-up SAFE algorithm.

Complete pre-diagnosis is a prerequisite for using the follow-up SAFE. This includes X-rays and corresponding sonographic findings from the initial situation. These are used later for comparison and diagnosis of a deviation. Exact documentation of the level and projection is essential for the reproduction of the findings.

20.4.7 Positioning

The positioning is individual and depends on the examination region. In general, the patient should be in a comfortable position with free access to the examination region. Splints should be removed completely. If this is not possible, an X-ray assessment should be preferred. Suboptimal solutions, for example, examinations with a cast, should be avoided.

If possible, hang the limb freely to allow adequate access with the transducer. Soft positioning aids for support are helpful.

20.4.8 Levels

At least three, if possible four leves must be documented. With metacarpal and metatarsal fractures, this can, for example, can be achieved by two oblique dorsal and two oblique volar projections. Even if the axial levels parallel to the shaft axis are the standard, transverse cuts can also be helpful for this indication; for example, in the case of long oblique or torsion fractures that are difficult to recognize in the longitudinal section (Figs. 20.5 and 20.6).

20.5 Examination

After the bone is shown as a bright, sharp line, the transducer is first aligned parallel to the longitudinal axis. This can be seen from the fact that the bone is shown across the entire

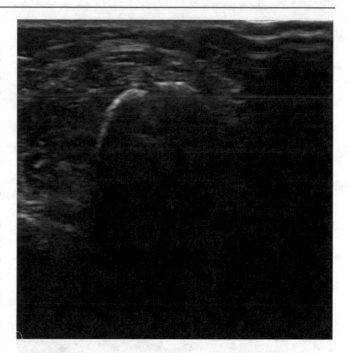

Fig. 20.5 Oblique fracture on the tibia; fracture gap in the transverse plane; the gap is difficult to see in the axial plane. (©Ackermann and Eckert 2015; Courtesy of off label media)

width of the image section. In the case of cross sections, the transducer is then turned through 90°.

To display longer sections, the cortex is scanned and documented in sections. The joints should also be mapped as defined endpoints.

20.6 Evaluation

The assessment is always made in comparison with the first (oldest) available finding from day 0, so as not to overlook slow deviations, in no case only the last finding is taken into account. A change in the bone axis and a widening of the fracture gap indicates a dislocation.

Intraosseous processes cannot be adequately assessed sonographically.

20.6.1 Examples

Figs. 20.7, 20.8, 20.9, 20.10, 20.11, 20.12, 20.13, and 20.14

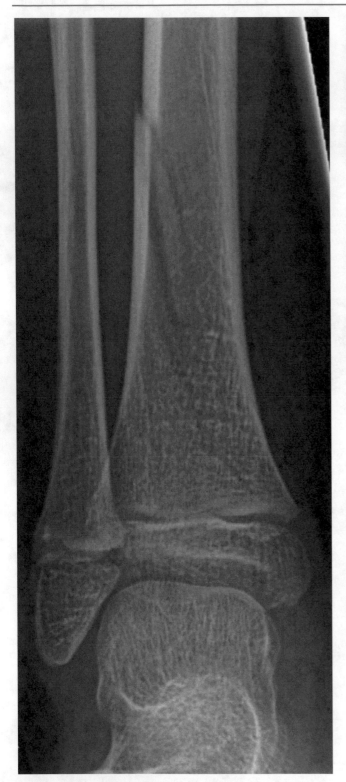

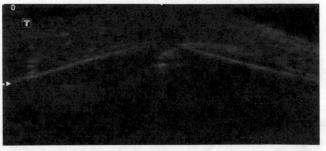

Fig. 20.7 Example 1 of a shaft fracture of a long bone in the middle of the shaft. (©Ackermann and Eckert 2015; Courtesy of off label media)

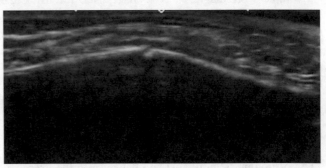

Fig. 20.8 Example 2 of a shaft fracture of a long bone in the middle of the shaft. (©Ackermann and Eckert 2015; Courtesy of off label media)

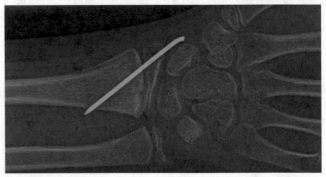

Fig. 20.9 Example 3a: wire osteosynthesis of a distal radius fracture (X-ray image). (©Ackermann and Eckert 2015; Courtesy of off label media)

Fig. 20.6 Same fracture as in Fig. 20.5. (©Ackermann and Eckert 2015; Courtesy of off label media)

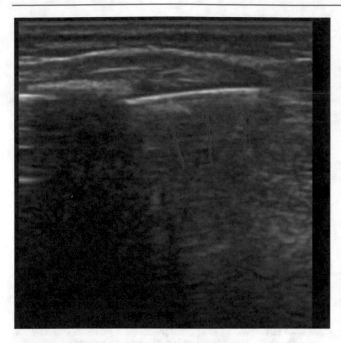

Fig. 20.10 Example 3b: ultrasound reflex of the K-wire. (©Ackermann and Eckert 2015; Courtesy of off label media)

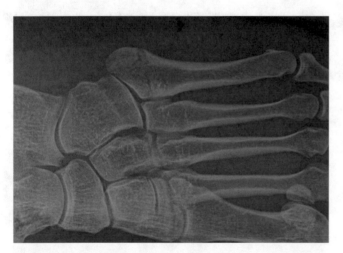

Fig. 20.11 Example 4a: MFK 5 basic fracture in an AP X-ray. (©Ackermann and Eckert 2015; Courtesy of off label media)

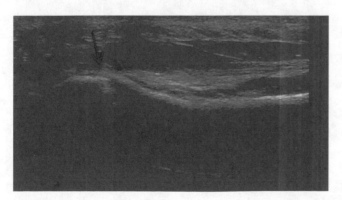

Fig. 20.12 Example 4b: MFK 5 fracture sonographic level dorsal. (©Ackermann and Eckert 2015; Courtesy of off label media)

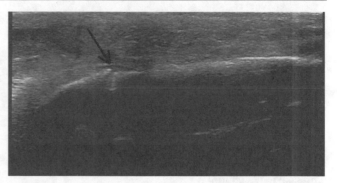

Fig. 20.13 Example 4c: MFK 5 lateral sonographic level fracture. (©Ackermann and Eckert 2015; Courtesy of off label media)

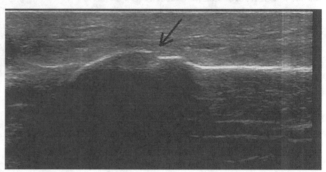

Fig. 20.14 Example 4d: MFK 5 fracture plantar sonographic level. (©Ackermann and Eckert 2015; Courtesy of off label media)

20.7 Diagnosis

Sonography for this indication only serves to exclude an undesirable course and not for a diagnosis. Therefore, if there is any suspicion of deviations, a radiological clarification is initiated and used for further therapy. There is currently insufficient experience with purely sonographic therapy control.

20.8 Pitfalls and Red Flags

20.8.1 Comparison with the Last Finding

For organizational reasons, it is often easier to use only the latest sonographic findings for comparison. However, the examiner can overlook slow changes. Therefore, the first finding that represents the reference must always be taken into account.

20.8.2 Documentation

Since there are no generally applicable standards for each individual bone, exact documentation of the patient, location, and projection is essential to ensure reproducibility. It is even more important with ultrasound than with X-ray diagnostics that findings can only be compared with the same projection, so they must be evident from the documentation and repeatable.

20.8.3 Increasing Pain

If the symptoms increase under adequate therapy, this is always a sign of a possible complication and gives reason for a precise reevaluation.

20.8.4 Infection and Material Failure

Questions regarding infection and osteosynthesis material cannot be answered adequately sonographically and are not the subject of the investigation.

20.8.5 Articular Fractures

With increasing experience and certainty, the examiner tends to also assess joint fractures sonographically. Here it is assumed that an identical position of the easily representable metaphysis implies an unchanged situation intra-articularly. Be warned. There is currently no conclusive evidence that justifies the use of sonography for joint fractures.

Further Reading

Axial Deviations Can Be Represented Well Sonographically

1. Grechenig W, Clement H, Schatz B, Klein A, Grechenig M. Sonographic fracture diagnostics-an experimental study-ultrasonographic diagnosis of fractures—an experimental study. Biomed Eng. 1997;42:138–45.

Ultrasound-Based Reduction of Fractures

2. Chinnock B, et al. Ultrasound-guided reduction of distal radius fractures. J Emerg Med. 2011;40(3):308–12.
3. Ang SH, Lee SW, Lam KY. Ultrasound-guided reduction of distal radius fractures. Am J Emerg Med. 2010;28(9):1002–8.

Shaft Fractures Can Be Visualized Very Well (Including Meta-analysis)

4. Chartier LB, Bosco L, Lapointe-Shaw L, Chenkin J. Use of point-of-care ultrasound in long bone fractures: a systematic review and meta-analysis. Can J Emerg Med. 2017;19(2):131–42.

Very Good Sensitivity for Ankle Fractures

5. Atilla OD, Yesilaras M, Kilic TY, Tur FC, Reisoglu A, Sever M, Aksay E. The accuracy of bedside ultrasonography as a diagnostic tool for fractures in the ankle and foot. Acad Emerg Med. 2014;21(9):1058–61.

Callus Display with Ultrasound

21

Christian Tesch

21.1 Synopsis

1.1 Rationale of application: X-ray-free direct representation of the connective tissue reaction in fracture healing in the six stages of all sonographically visible bones, mainly in the shaft area.

1.2 Level of evidence: IIa.

1.3 Indication: For monitoring the course of all secondary healing fractures that are visible on ultrasound and in which the cortex can be displayed safely. Especially in the transition from the inflammation to the repair phase of the secondary fracture healing (see Secondary Fracture Healing) there is a reliable assessment of the fracture healing about 2 weeks before the X-ray, which can be omited.

1.4 Age of the patient: Every age.

1.5 Contraindication: None since ultrasound is only used to assess fracture healing. Open fractures can also be assessed sonographically using sterile coatings.

1.6 Examination: Visualisation of the fracture in at least two levels, in the case of shaft fractures, ultrasound must be made in four levels along the length of the long bones (alternatively on the forearm in three levels).

1.7 Indications for additional X-ray diagnostics: If the fracture is suspected, X-rays should be taken. In the case of delayed fracture healing and nonunion (see p. 11), a CT examination should prove the missing or partial expansion in the cancellous and/or cortical area.

1.8 Pitfalls: Joint fractures show no callus formation in the sense of the stage classification according to Ricciardi.

1.9 Red flags: Infection signs should prompt immediately further measures (laboratory control, X-ray control, magnetic resonance imaging, scintigraphy) if necessary.

21.2 History

Taken from the work of Ricciardi from 1992 [1, 2] with ultrasound devices with a very low resolution at the time (Fig. 21.1):

Together with his coauthors, the latter created a basis with which one could follow the callus distraction well [3] and, based on these findings, created a system for the representation of callus formation.

Even today, the use of this division of the healing stages, which the authors checked, is helpful. With this simple method, an almost microscopic assessment of the fracture stages is possible with our high-resolution devices of today.

Trauma surgeons appreciate the ability to recognize the point in time of axial resilience as early as possible so that they can release the pressure and tensile loads that are so important for fracture stabilization. In addition, the correct fracture healing can be observed in the further course, and abnormalities can be recognized immediately.

Chachan published an article in 2015 in which he asked whether the ultrasound examination of fracture healing would have brought the end of the X-ray follow-up [4]? This provocation of the conventional diagnosis of fractures is at least worth considering, because the fracture gap is open for a long time, especially in intramedullary osteosynthesis procedures, which is why X-rays are taken at short intervals, on which one can hardly see any changes. The authors convincingly describe which signs of normal fracture healing can be seen on ultrasound, making an X-ray image unnecessary at

C. Tesch (✉)
Praxis für Orthopädie und Chirurgie, Hamburg, Germany
e-mail: christian@gelenktesch.de

© Springer Nature Switzerland AG 2021
O. Ackermann (ed.), *Fracture Sonography*, https://doi.org/10.1007/978-3-030-63839-9_21

139

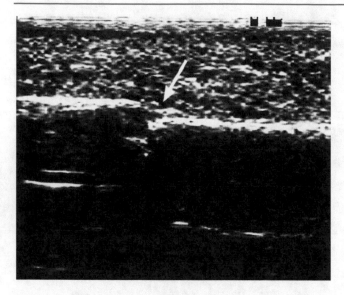

Fig. 21.1 Ultrasound image of a stage 2 fracture, taken in 1995, the arrow points to the fracture gap, the reverberation artifacts are interrupted, a fracture hematoma cannot be seen here, and the resolution is very low. (From Tesch 2018a; Courtesy of Seminar-Label-Media)

Table 21.1 Classification of the stages [1, 2]

Stage	Days	Signs
1	0–10	Fracture gap with hematoma *Fracture ends sharply defined, the gap can be traced in depth*
2	11–19	Smear the ends of the fractures *a collar forms at the ends of the fractures*
3	20–35	Bridge callus *The collars approach each other and form an echo-rich bridge* *No sound shadow behind the callus*
4	36–49	Mineralization begins *Sound shadow behind the callus*
5	50–89	Callus mineralization *Reverberation artifacts interrupted*
6	90–140	Callus remodeling *Reverberation artifacts no longer interrupted*

this point. They note that ultrasound can show the fracture consolidates on average 3 weeks before the X-ray.

The problem of delayed fracture healing can be easily solved with the help of ultrasound diagnostics; the examiner only has to map the fracture gap in the course and compare it with the defined stages. As soon as stage 3 according to Ricciardi is reached (formation of the bridging callus, see Table 21.1), the tensile and the compressive load can be started because only plastic deformation is now possible. When stage 4 (beginning mineralization) is reached, the load can be increased to such an extent that bending and torsional loads can also be released (see Table 21.1).

Healing begins with the injury, it is controlled vegetatively and in a humoral manner. Bone fracture healing takes place primarily (direct sprouting of the osteons with direct firm contact of the fracture ends) or secondary (the fracture ends have minimal relative movements). The following is only about secondary fracture healing.

21.3   Secondary Fracture Healing

The following osteological principles for secondary fracture healing are important for understanding further explanations [5]:

(a) Bone is subject to a constant remodeling process, which is controlled vegetatively and in a humoral manner.
(b) Bone is a quasi-brittle material that absorbs energy through the formation of microcracks ("micro-cracks" and sub lamellar damage (cracks <1 μm)).
(c) Microcracks have a length of 50–100 μm, were already described in 1960 [6] and are the "engine" of fracture healing or remodeling due to apoptosis of osteocytes.

Fracture healing takes place in three phases, based on the phases in inflammation teaching, founded by Celsus (in 20) and Galen (in 180) with the signs Rubor, Tumor, Calor, Dolor, and Functio laesa:

First inflammation phase (day 0–ca.20).

(a) Immigration of monocytes, granulocytes, and histiocytes into the fracture hematoma.
(b) Release of histamine and cytokines increases periosteal blood flow.
(c) Osteoblastic cell differentiation.
(d) Phagocytosis and vascular sprout.

Second reparation phase (day 21 to 12th week).

(a) Formation of cell-rich granulation tissue with fibroblasts, osteoblasts, and macrophages.
(b) Formation of collagen type I matrix promoted.
(c) Callus is mineralized.
(d) Callus is hardened and rebuilt into poorly organized braided bones.
(e) This creates biomechanically firm bones.

Third conversion phase (13 weeks to 12th month).

(a) The poorly ordered braided bone is converted into stable, highly structured lamella bones with Havers

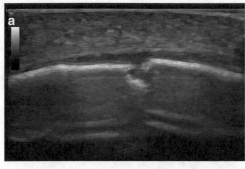 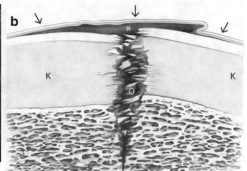

Fig. 21.2 (**a**) Sonographic image of a fracture in stage 1 (fracture gap with hematoma), the sharply depicted fracture ends and the hypoechoic zone above the fracture ends, which represent the hematoma, can be seen. (From Tesch 2018a; Courtesy of Seminar-Label-Media). (**b**)

Schematic drawing showing the cortex (K), the raised periosteum (↓), the clearly visible fracture gap (o), the reverberation artifacts (<), and the hematoma (*)

and Volkmann canal systems according to the stress zones.

(b) Absorption of excess callus leads to the original geometry of the bone.

21.4 Stages of Fracture Healing

Morphologically, fibrinous entanglement of the blood clot occurs in the inflammation phase with completed blood coagulation, and thus, the crosslinking of the hematoma. After the fibrin threads have been adequately cross-linked, the vessels are sprouted in order to ensure the blood supply and to form collagen fibers in order to stabilize the fixation callus. These vessels can also be visualized sonographically in the powerdoppler mode [7]. The transition to the repair phase, in which the bridge callus, which is essential for stabilization, can be formed by mineralization, is fluid. These processes can be observed sonographically. The work of the two colleagues Ricciardi and Perisinotto has observed and systematized the changes in the region of the fracture cleft after surgery in patients with an external fixator. The original information on the timing of the stadiums is related to the time of the operation. These times are modified in the following explanations.

21.4.1 Stage 1, Day 0–10

The representation in the ultrasound image focuses on the correct representation of the fracture ends. These should be taken orthogonally, which is achieved with the sharpest

image of the anterior edge of the cortex (see Fig. 21.2). This principle is always the same, the sharpest image of the cortex is therefore a basic condition. Ideally, the gray values should always be set the same, this can be done with a good preset of the transducer, which should always be called up before the examination. The examination conditions should also always be the same from the lighting conditions.

The characteristics at this stage are the sharp edges of the fracture ends and the inhomogeneous, hypoechoic zone above the fracture, which represent the hematoma. Typically, the reverberation artifacts are interrupted in-depth, which is important in order to detect almost undisplaced fractures or stress fractures.

21.4.2 Stage 2, Days 11–19

The previously sharp image of the fracture ends and gradually blurs, small echo-rich structures (collars) form at the fracture ends. These echo-rich structures correspond to periosteal callus formation. The characteristics at this stage are the connective tissue changes in the sense of an intensive cross-linking of the collagen network. An echo-poor zone spanning everything can be seen above the echo-rich structure in the fracture area (Fig. 21.3).

21.4.3 Stage 3, Days 20–35

In this phase, the initial callus is increasingly mineralized, which is shown by an increase in the echo-rich structures in the fracture gap. The echo-rich bridge is still irregularly lim-

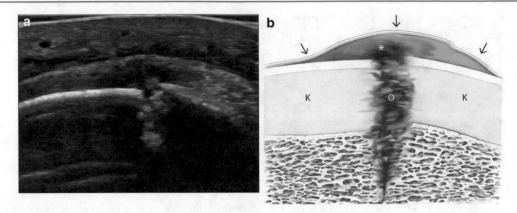

Fig. 21.3 (**a**) Sonographic image of a fracture in stage 2 (initial callus), showing the further apart fracture ends and the formation of the collar there (From Tesch 2018a; Courtesy of Seminar-Label-Media).

(**b**) Schematic drawing showing the widening fracture gap (o) and the formation of the collar with the initial callus (*), the periosteum has risen further (↓) over the fracture area an anechoic zone has formed

Fig. 21.4 (**a**) Sonographic image of a fracture in stage 3 (bridge callus), the echo-rich structures above the fracture gap and the view into it can be seen (From Tesch 2018a; Courtesy of Seminar-Label-Media). (**b**) Schematic drawing of the fracture with the cortex (K) and the echo-rich bridge (↓) and the low-echo zone over the fracture area

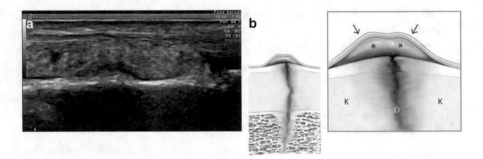

ited. As in stage 2, the fracture gap can be viewed without any problems. For the first time, these structures would also be visible in the X-ray image.

This phase is important for the further development of the treatment because either the fracture is now stabilized or the bone remains in the phase of an extended bone fracture healing in the worst case of nonunion. The hypoechoic zone above the fracture can still be seen (Fig. 21.4).

21.4.4 Stage 4, Days 36–49)

The echo-rich structures in the fracture gap become more homogeneous and smoother, which is accompanied by the formation of a sound shadow as an expression of increasing mineralization. The fracture is now also stable and could only be separated by gross force. The hypoechoic zone above the fracture can still be seen. Reverberation artifacts cannot be identified with certainty (Fig. 21.5).

21.4.5 Stage 5, Days 50–89

The callus is now increasingly calcified, the hypoechoic zone over the fracture disappears. The reverberation artifacts are vis-

ible again, but are interrupted by the sound shadow of the echo-rich bridge. The cortex reflex becomes smoother (Fig. 21.6).

21.4.6 Stage 6, Days 90–140

The cortex reflex is clearly visible and the reverberation artifacts are no longer interrupted. During this time, the callus is modeled, the excess shape is leveled, and the cortex is adjusted in thickness according to the strength requirements (Fig. 21.7).

21.4.6.1 Indications and Patient Age

The method was developed by the first descriptors in order to observe the late or invisible callus formation in intramedullary nail and external fixator osteosynthesis. Accordingly, it is used to monitor and document the stages of fracture healing through callus imaging; applicable in every patient age.

All fractures of bones visible for ultrasound are suitable, especially fractures of long bones (fractures in these bones also represent the majority of the problematic fractures). Open fractures can also be examined using sterile transducer covers. The method is ideal for fractures treated with external fixators. Joint fractures usually do not show any visible callus formation.

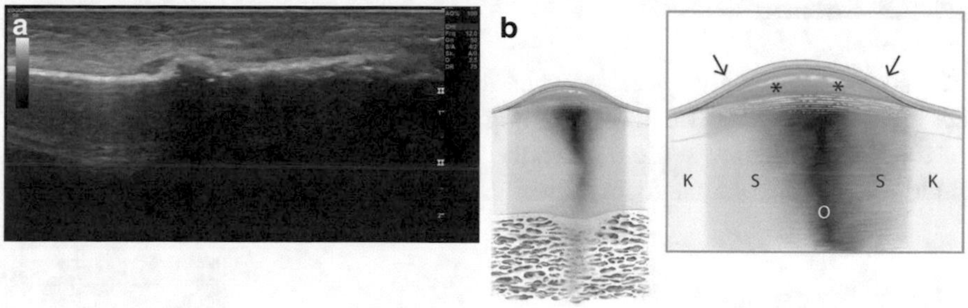

Fig. 21.5 (**a**) Sonographic image of a fracture in stage 4 (beginning mineralization), the echo-rich bridge with the acoustic shadow behind it can be seen (From Tesch 2018a; Courtesy of Seminar-Label-Media). (**b**) Schematic drawing with the the fracture in stage 4 with mineralized echorich bridge (blue with*), above periosteum (*Pfeil nach unten*). Fracture gap not seen and visible mineralized callus with shadow (S), corticalis (K)

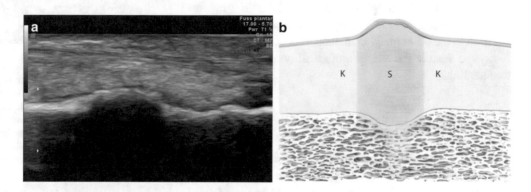

Fig. 21.6 (**a**) Sonographic image of a fracture in stage 5 (callus calcification), the acoustic shadow of the echo-rich bridge can be seen, the artifacts of the reverberation are interrupted by the shadow, (From Tesch 2018a; Courtesy of Seminar-Label-Media) (**b**) Scheme of the fracture at the stage of mineralization, stage 5, days 50–89

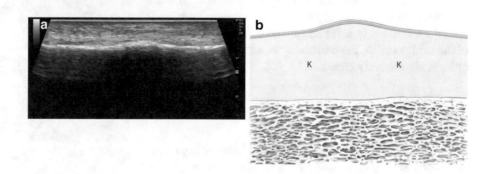

Fig. 21.7 (**a**) Sonographic image of a fracture in stage 6 (callus remodeling) can be seen (From Tesch 2018a; Courtesy of Seminar-Label-Media). (**b**) Scheme of the fracture at the stage of callus remodeling, stage 62, days 90–140

21.4.6.2   Contraindications and Indications for X-ray Diagnostics

Primarily healing fractures show no callus formation, for example, in plate osteosynthesis. Here, ultrasound diagnostics can only be used for secondary problems (fixation of tendons, loosening, and protrusion of the screws). X-ray diagnosis is always necessary to prove the correct position of the fracture, the osteosynthesis, or the dislocation.

21.5   Examination

21.5.1   Positioning

Comfortable supine or prone positioning (examination of the dorsal tibia, fibula, and femur region).

A linear transducer with an frequency of 12 MHz is suitable for examining the fracture hematoma and callus. For special images in higher resolution, transducers with 16 MHz (matrix transducer) or with 18 MHz (hockey stick transducer) should be used. With this transducer selection, all structures in the near field can be mapped well. For deeper bones (femur, femoral neck, dorsal tibia, plantar metatarsalia, we need a low-frequency transducer with 9 MHz.

21.5.2 Levels

It is preferably examined in the longitudinal direction of the bone. Four views are required to assess the entire limb.

21.5.3 Setting

The correct setting always arises when the cortical reflex is set most sharply, then we have an orthograde representation of the bone. It makes sense to have the fracture gap in the middle of the picture, the focus there.

21.5.4 Assessment

Fracture sonography for assessing fracture healing has a great advantage that it is quickly available and has no radiation exposure. It depicts the soft tissue analogously to magnetic resonance imaging. Liquids are black to gray on ultrasound, white to gray in magnetic resonance imaging. In addition to the other imaging method, it is excellent for using X-rays to answer the question of stability and regular fracture healing.

21.5.5 Diagnosis, Controls

The important point in time at the end of the inflammation phase at the transition to the repair phase (see secondary fracture healing) sets the course for regular bone consolidation or delayed fracture healing or even "nonunion" [8]. We can prove this with the ultrasound examination in stage 2 with the transition to 3. If there are no signs of the formation of the bridge callus, the probability of a fracture healing disorder is significantly increased [9, 10].

21.5.6 Therapy

Accordingly, the therapy can be conducted based solely on the ultrasound examination, in which the usual increase in stress is suspended until the signs of stage 3 of fracture healing become visible or measures are taken to exert therapeutic influence on fracture healing (e.g., shock wave or ultrasound therapy).

In the case of delayed fracture healing, we do not see a transition to stage 3 on ultrasound; the echo-rich bridge is not formed. No other examination method can reliably detect this simple sign and help to control further therapy.

Example: with the reliable detection of the lack of fracture healing (see Fig. 21.8), the therapeutic measures (shock wave) described above were taken to stimulate fracture healing.

21.6   Pitfalls and Red Flags

This procedure basically applies to all fractures. In intra-articular fractures, however, callus formation is difficult or not to be observed (femoral head and neck fractures (see Fig. 21.9)

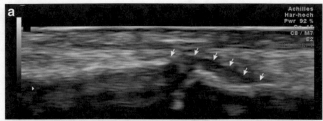
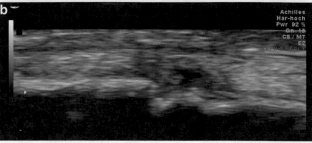

Fig. 21.8 (**a**) Sonography of a metatarsal osteotomy, echo-rich reflexes are missing in the area of the fracture gap as a sign of mineralization of the callus, the fracture gap is deeply visible. The ends of the fractures have a relative movement and (←) indicate the connective tissue fixation of the fracture. (**b**) The same region 4 months later after 10×0.4 mJ/mm^2 shock wave therapy no longer shows an insight into the fracture gap, the fracture ends no longer move against each other and a deepening through the CT is detectable (From Tesch 2018a; Courtesy of Seminar-Label-Media)

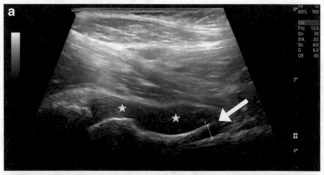
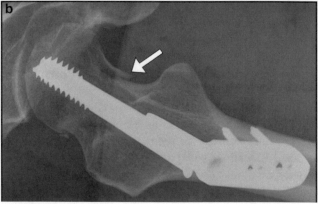

Fig. 21.9 (**a**) Sonography of the femoral head and neck fracture, the callus was not observed as described during the entire observation period; sonography did not show any effusion over the entire observation period, while joint capsule (*) is very thickend. The fracture (←) is seen in the sonographic image exactly like in the X-ray image. (**b**) X-ray image of the fracture, which was primarily treated with a dynamic hip screw, note the exact match of the fracture (←) in the Lauenstein projection for sonography. (From Tesch 2018a; Courtesy of Seminar-Label-Media)

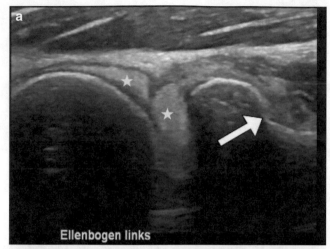

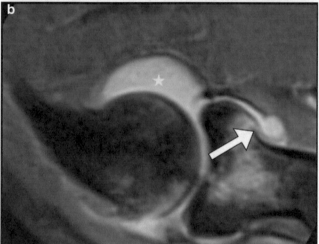

Fig. 21.10 (**a**) Sonography of the radial head fracture, this was primarily overlooked, diagnosis by ultrasound, here you can see an articular effusion (*), in the area of the fracture (→) there is no initial callus as described (see Table 21.1). (**b**) Magnetic resonance imaging, which was carried out for the exact classification of the fracture, shows exactly the same finding, the joint effusion (*) and the fracture (→) (From Tesch 2018a; Courtesy of Seminar-Label-Media)

and the same in radius head fractures (see Fig. 21.10)). The reason is probably to be found in the constant movement of the fracture in the fluid joint environment. Here, attention must be paid to the unchanged fracture position and the relative movement of the fracture ends. In addition, ultrasound can identify or rule out joint effusion (see Figs. 21.9 and 21.10).

Failure to heal fractures (stage 2 does not change to 3) should primarily lead to frequent checks, an infection should always be considered, which then leads to the laboratory and magnetic resonance imaging check. In the later stages of failure to heal a fracture, a CT must be done.

21.7 Conclusion for Practice

The assessment of the morphology of the fracture healing stages enables the examiner to use a simple means to display the callus much more precisely than with X-ray; as a rough rule, the callus is visible on ultrasound 2–3 weeks before X-ray detection. This has made it possible to control the therapy without having to use complex procedures such as magnetic resonance imaging and scintigraphy.

References

1. Ricciardi L, Perissinotto A, Dabala M. External callus development on ultrasound and its mechanical correlation. Ital J Orthop Traumatol. 1992;18:223–9.
2. Ricciardi L, Perissinotto A, Dabala M. Mechanical monitoring of fracture healing using ultrasound imaging. Clin Orthop. 1993;293:71–6.
3. Ricciardi L, Perissinotto A, Visentin E. Ultrasonography in the evaluation of osteogenesis in fractures treated with Hoffmann external fixation. Ital J Orthop Traumatol. 1986;12(2):185–9.
4. Chachan S, Tudu B, Sahu B. Ultrasound monitoring of fracture healing: is this the end of radiography in fracture follow-ups? J Orthop Trauma. 2015;29(3):e133–8. https://doi.org/10.1097/BOT.0000000000000207.
5. Kurth A, Lange U. Fachwissen Osteologie. München: Elsevier; 2018.
6. Frost HM. Presence of microscopic cracks in vivo in bone. Henry Ford Hosp Med Bull. 1960;8:9.
7. Drakonaki EE, Garbi A. Metatarsal stress fracture diagnosed with high-resolution sonography. J Ultrasound Med. 2010;29(3):473–6. doi: 29/3/473 [pii].
8. DePalma AF. Repair of fractures. In: DePalma AF (Hrsg). The management of fractures and dislocations an atlas, vol. 1. 2 Aufl. Philadelphia: W B Saunders Company; 1970. S10–S14.
9. Bica D, Sprouse RA, Armen J. Diagnosis and management of common foot fractures. Am Fam Physician. 2016;93(3):183–91. doi: d12379 [pii]
10. Csongradi JJ, Maloney WJ. Ununited lower limb fractures. West J Med. 1989;150(6):675–80.

Nonunions

22

Christian Fischer

22.1 Synopsis

1.1 Clinical relevance: early, perfusion-based detection of an unphysiological fracture healing and identification of infected nonunions.

1.2 Level of evidence: III.

1.3 Indication: preoperative infection diagnosis and postoperative monitoring of the healing process.

1.4 Contraindications regarding the use of contrast agents: right–left shunts, severe pulmonary hypertension, uncontrolled systemic hypertension, acute respiratory distress syndrome, hypersensitivity or allergic to the contrast agent.

1.5 Examination: longitudinal plane, assessment of the fracture or nonunion in the area with the largest gap width, video recording after application of contrast medium.

1.6 Quantification of perfusion: software-supported using regions of interest, time–intensity curves and perfusion parameters.

22.2 Introduction

As a result of delayed or impaired fracture healing, 5–10% of all fractures develop into a nonunion [1]. Considering the numerous revision surgeries with repeated hospitalization, their treatment tends to be tedious, time-consuming, and cost-intensive, especially if the therapy is uncertain [2, 3]. Efficient treatment of nonunion requires diagnostic tools that provide therapeutic and prognostic information at an early stage, such as regarding the presence of an infection or poor blood circulation and thereby set the course for a consequent adaptation of the therapy.

Recently, the use of contrast-enhanced ultrasound (CEUS) demonstrated promising results in the healing prediction and classification of infected nonunions. CEUS enables an assessment of local tissue perfusion [4, 5], which is a crucial factor in bone metabolism and the process of bone regeneration [6, 7]. From a functional point of view, CEUS is, therefore, able to assess the microperfusion as a respective surrogate parameter, and can detect pathological changes at an early stage. This would not be feasible using conventional fracture and nonunion diagnostic tools like X-ray and computed tomography.

The ultrasound contrast agent applied in CEUS examinations contains small microbubbles consisting of a sulfur hexafluoride gas core enclosed by a stabilizing phospholipid shell [8]. After intravenous injection, they distribute throughout the vascular system and allow for an assessment of the perfusion in real time, even at the level of capillary vessels [5]. In contrast to MRI contrast agents, which are subject to rapid extravasation, ultrasound contrast agents act as purely intravascular marker substances [4, 9] until they are eventually exhaled via the lungs [5]. Through specific interactions of the microbubbles, with the ultrasonic waves, an amplified signal (compared to the surrounding tissue) is generated, which directly reflects the local microperfusion of the examined section. These signal changes can then be quantified using dedicated software [5, 10, 11].

Initially, CEUS was exclusively established for the diagnosis of liver and kidney lesions, but its usage has recently expanded to the field of musculoskeletal indications [10, 12]. Numerous current studies analyze the applicability of CEUS for the diagnosis of fractures and nonunions. The focus of these investigations lies on the microperfusion within the fracture or nonunion gap, which can be measured perioperatively using CEUS.

Furthermore, it could be demonstrated that the fracture callus presents physiological perfusion in tibial fractures that heal in a timely manner (Figs. 22.1 and 22.2), while atrophic tibial nonunions showed particularly low, and infected tibial

C. Fischer (✉)
Universitätsklinikum Heidelberg, Zentrum für Orthopädie, Unfallchirurgie und, Paraplegiologie, Heidelberg, Germany
e-mail: christian.fischer@med.uni-heidelberg.de

© Springer Nature Switzerland AG 2021
O. Ackermann (ed.), *Fracture Sonography*, https://doi.org/10.1007/978-3-030-63839-9_22

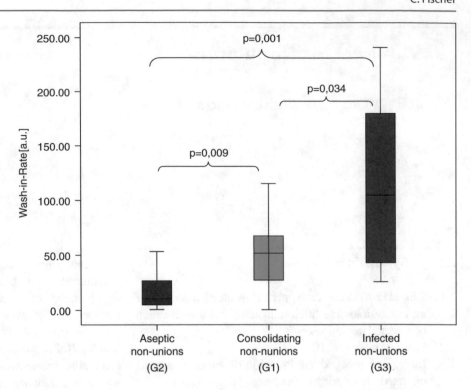

Fig. 22.1 Boxplots of wash-in-rates demonstrating the microperfusion within the fracture and nonunion gap. Comparison of microperfusion between consolidating fractures and (G1) aseptic (G2) or infected (G3) nonunions. (a.u. = arbitrary units). (Courtesy of Fischer et al. 2018)

nonunions excessive levels of perfusion [13, 14]. Normal bone regeneration, therefore, appears to be associated with physiological perfusion, the upward and downward deviation from which should make the examiner aware of the possible implied conditions above.

Until now, infected nonunions could not be reliably detected preoperatively or intraoperatively due to their predominantly chronic nature and clinical in appearance, that is, without classic signs of inflammation such as rubor, calor, or tumor. The use of conventional imaging methods (X-ray, computed tomography) as well as the laboratory parameters CRP and leucocytes are not reliable in this context either. In aseptic nonunions, CRP levels may controversially even be higher than in infected ones [13]. Osseous microperfusion appears to be more sensitive in the detection of infections: based on perfusion measurements in the nonunion gap, CEUS shows a significantly higher blood flow in infected, compared to aseptic nonunions and can thus reveal existing infections even before planned revision surgery [13], which is therapeutically highly relevant: infected nonunions require an advanced treatment according to a multistage strategy, that is, according to the Masquelet technique. Furthermore, nonunions, which are preoperatively identified as aseptic by CEUS, could be treated in one single surgical intervention with the direct insertion of the bone graft and reosteosynthesis [13, 15].

The consolidation process after revision surgery of a nonunion extends over a significantly longer period than with ordinary fractures [15, 16]. Thus, imaging methods conventionally used (X-ray, computed tomography), which purely rely on morphological changes (Fig. 22.3), can only provide delayed information on whether the nonunion actually heals or not [15–17]. This is problematic in cases of a delayed con-

solidation, where the indication for the revision surgery should be given as early as possible. In addition to the previously described infection-related preoperative hyperperfusion, diminished perfusion with deficient consolidation must be distinguished from the physiological blood flow in a healing fracture or nonunion, as recent studies demonstrate (Figs. 22.1 and 22.2).

Corresponding to this, our data suggest that a conclusion regarding the probability of consolidation can be made as early as 12 weeks after the revision surgery, based on the individual microperfusion [14] assessed by CEUS (Figs. 22.4 and 22.5).

If there is no prospect of successful consolidation, an earlier intervention would be possible.

Dynamic contrast-enhanced magnetic resonance imaging (DCE-MRI), which can also be used to measure perfusion in the nonunion gap, demonstrates a comparable potential regarding a prognostic quality in fracture healing [13, 16]. However, DCE-MRI is inferior to CEUS in terms of cost, contrast agent tolerance, and its susceptibility to implant-associated artifacts [4, 11].

22.3 Indication

Recent findings suggest the following indications for the use of CEUS in cases of delayed fracture healing and nonunions:

- Planned revision surgery due to a possible underlying infection.
- Prediction and monitoring of the consolidation in the postoperative course after revision.

Fig. 22.2 X-ray imaging of an aseptic (**a**) and infected (**c**) nonunion as well as a consolidating tibial fracture (**b**) in two planes. Assessment of the corresponding nonunion and fracture gap using B-mode sonography (**d–f**). These images are correlated with their respective CEUS-based time–intensity curves (**g–i**) after software-assisted quantification. Significant deviations in perfusion were evident between infected (red) and atrophic (blue) compared to physiological (green) fracture healing. (Courtesy of Fischer et al. 2018)

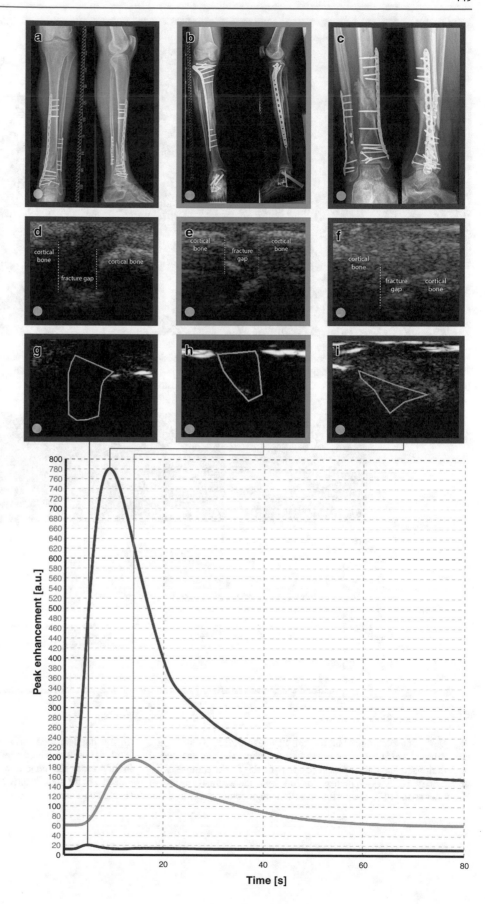

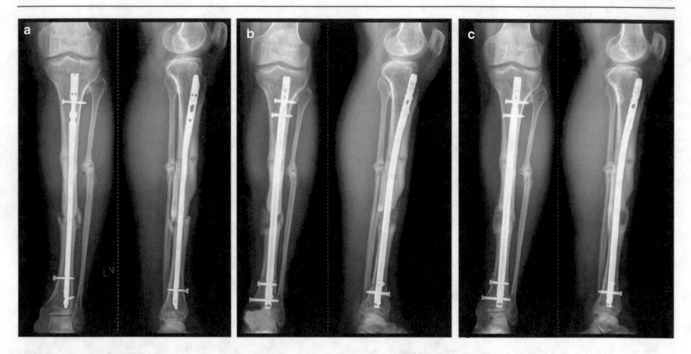

Fig. 22.3 X-ray imaging of a consolidating nonunion before revision surgery (**a**), 12 weeks postoperative (**b**), and 52 weeks postoperative (**c**). A CEUS-based perfusion assessment performed 12 weeks postoperatively predicted the eventual consolidation of the nonunion. (Courtesy of Krammer et al. [14])

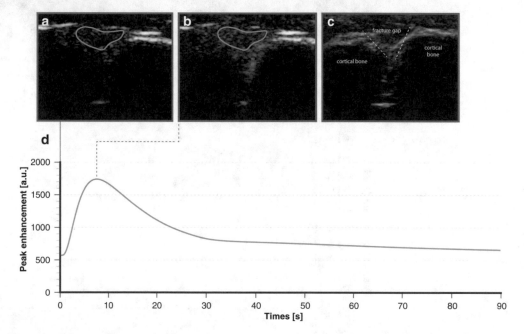

Fig. 22.4 Consolidating tibial fracture 12 weeks after revision surgery. CEUS-based perfusion assessment before bolus injection (**a**) and at peak contrast agent enhancement (**b**). In B-mode (**c**), the conture of the nonunion gap is assessed in its maximum depth and width. (Courtesy of Krammer et al. [14]). The perfusion within the nonunion gap was quantified using dedicated software, and time–intensity curves were calculated (**d**) based on the manually selected regions of interest (green line). In this case, the nonunion eventually consolidated, which is also reflected in the significantly higher gap perfusion, compared to the persisting non-unions displayed in Fig. 22.5. (a.u. = arbitrary units)

Fig. 22.5 Persisting nonunions 12 weeks after revision surgery. CEUS-based perfusion assessment before bolus injection (**a**) and at peak contrast agent enhancement (**b**). In B-mode (**c**), the conture of the nonunion gap is assessed in its maximum depth and width. The perfusion within the nonunion gap was quantified using dedicated software, and time–intensity curves were calculated (**d**) based on the manually selected regions of interest (green line). (a.u. = arbitrary units). (Courtesy of Krammer et al. [14])

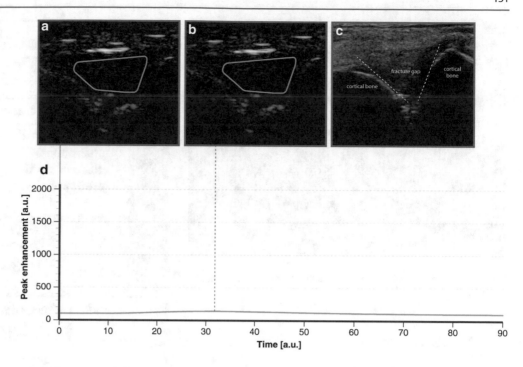

22.4 Contraindications

Considering CEUS as a contrast-agent based imaging modality, possible contraindications against these agents have to be taken into account. In general, ultrasound contrast agents are characterized by their good safety profile [18], which also applies for SonoVue©—an ultrasound contrast agent of the second generation [19], which is commonly used in Europe for CEUS examinations:

Adverse effects are extremely rare [18, 19]. The few existing contraindications include acute respiratory distress syndrome, right–left shunts, severe pulmonary and uncontrolled systemic hypertension, and an existing hypersensitivity to the active substance (see specialist information). Unlike conventional contrast-agent based imaging methods, no laboratory tests are necessary to assess liver and kidney function prior to the application [18].

22.5 Examination

The CEUS-based perfusion analysis should be standardized in order to compare the results generated. Accordingly, the settings of crucial, yet often device-specific functions (overall gain, focus, depth, mechanical index) have to be matched and selected identically in sequential examinations. The contrast agent is usually injected as a bolus (1.2–4.8 mL SonoVue©) via a peripheral intravenous cannula and subsequent flushing with 10 mL of saline solution via a three-way valve.

22.5.1 Setup

The optimal positioning of the patient depends on the location of the nonunion: the upper extremity is usually examined while sitting, while nonunions of the femur or tibia while lying. It is advisable to position the ultrasound device in such a way that both the examiner and the patient have a good view of the monitor in order to actively involve the patient in the examination process.

22.5.2 Sections and Planes

The bone should be examined using a linear transducer under light pressure. The aim is to represent the nonunion gap as broadly and deeply as possible without overlays or compromising the perfusion due to excess pressure. The cortical bone should be visible on both sides of the nonunion gap. The best way to achieve this is to "approach" the ideal ultrasound plane step by step:

By moving the transducer cranially and caudally, the gap is set in the center of the image. Proceeding from this, moving medially and laterally enables the display of the largest gap area.

If the transducer is tilted in this position, adjacent areas of the cortex can be sharply depicted. Turning the transducer is recommended for further optimization (e.g., the depth of the gap). The picture now set should be carefully labeled and referenced so that the same area can be reassessed during the course of follow-up checks.

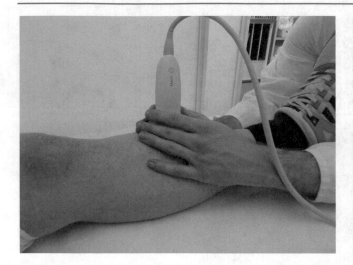

Fig. 22.6 Handling and stabilization of the ultrasound probe during the video recording

22.5.3 Overall Process

An assistant is required for the examination.

First, the nonunion gap is examined to its greatest extent in B-mode (5.2). The contrast mode is then selected; if preliminary examinations have already been carried out, the overall gain, focus, depth, and mechanical index are set analogously to these. The examiner saves the image as a reference.

In the next part of the examination, the main task of the examiner is to hold the transducer in a fixed position during the entire video recording of the nonunion gap that is now set in order to avoid movement artifacts. For this purpose, the examiner encloses the transducer with both hands, which he supports on the patient at the same time (Fig. 22.6).

The assistant involved carries out all further steps:

After switching to dual-image mode, the nonunion gap can be assessed in both B-mode and contrast mode. The special contrast mode with its low mechanical index ensures that the contrasted tissue is visualized without destroying the microbubbles. The patient is instructed not to move for the next 90 seconds of the video recording. As soon as the assistant starts the video recording, the contrast agent and the saline solution must be applied quickly in sequence. A few seconds later, the perfusion signal increases on the monitor in contrast-medium specific color signals, which the examiner can already assess qualitatively. However, the examiner and patient still must not move until the video ends to also adequately measure the agent's outflow kinetics.

22.6   Quantification and Assessment

Dedicated quantification programs (e.g., VueBox©, Bracco, Milan, Italy) are used to assess the CEUS sequences.

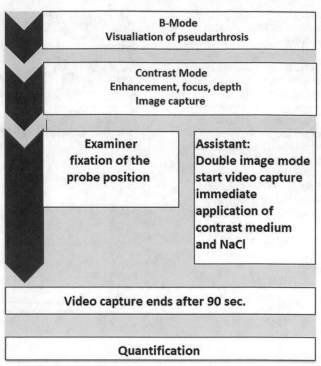

Fig. 22.7 User manual for VueBox© version 6.0 [http://www.contrastultrasound-modality.com/quantification-software/support/user-manual]. (Copyright© 2015 Bracco Suisse SA)

A so-called region of Interest (ROI) is placed in the nonunion gap by the examiner, strictly avoiding distortions of the perfusion measurement by surrounding structures such as arteries or fascia (Fig. 22.7).

Time–intensity curves can now be generated and various perfusion parameters calculated (Fig. 22.8). These include:

- Wash-in rate (WiR).
- Wash-in area under the curve (WiAUC).

Time to peak (TTP).

- Rise time (RT).
- Wash-in Perfusion Index (WiPI = WiAUC/RT).
- Wash-out Rate (WoR).
- Wash-out area under the curve (WoAUC)fall time (FT).

According to our study results, hyperperfusion shows an infection before revision surgery, whereas hypoperfusion indicates a lack of consolidation due to insufficient vascularization. To enable a clear interpretation of the individual perfusion kinetics of examined patients, cutoff values for the perfusion parameters must be defined. Figures 22.9 and 22.10 are examples of the ROC (Receiver Operating Characteristic) analyzes of two perfusion parameters (WiPI, WiR), from which the determined cutoff values can be calculated.

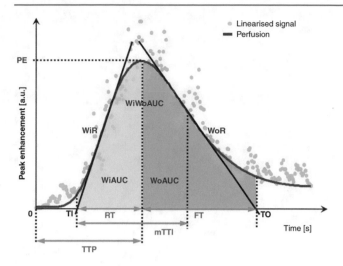

Fig. 22.8 A time–intensity curve (TIC) reflects the contrast agent kinetics after software quantification. Relevant parameters during the inflow phase are: WiR [a.u.], WiAUC [a.u.], TTP [s], RT [s]. The outflow kinetics are described by the parameters WoR [a.u.], WoAUC [a.u.], and FT [s]

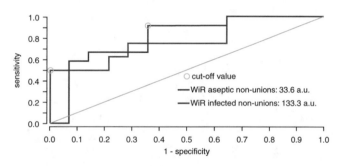

Fig. 22.9 Receiver operating characteristic (ROC) curves. A demonstration of the accuracy at which CEUS is able to differentiate between aseptic and infected nonunions. The calculated cutoff value for the wash-in rate (WiR) of aseptic nonunions was 33.6, compared to 136.3 in infected ones. (Courtesy of Fisher et al. 2018)

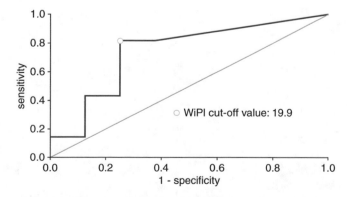

Fig. 22.10 Receiver operating characteristic (ROC) curve. Evaluation of CEUS-based Wash-in Perfusion Index (WiPI) for the prediction of eventual consolidation 12 weeks after revision surgery resulted in an optimal cutoff value of 19.9. (Courtesy of Krammer et al. [14])

However, since these values are based on pilot studies with a medium number of cases, they should be regarded as provisional. The establishment of generally applicable cutoff values will be carried out in the context of further, more extensive studies.

In summary, dynamic CEUS proves to be a diagnostically valuable tool, which can support the diagnosis and therapy decisions of fractures and nonunions in the future.

References

1. Tzioupis C, Giannoudis PV. Prevalence of long-bone non-unions. Injury. 2007;38(Suppl 2):S3–9.
2. Antonova E, et al. Tibia shaft fractures: costly burden of nonunions. BMC Musculoskelet Disord. 2013;14:42.
3. Brinker MR, et al. The devastating effects of tibial non-union on health-related quality of life. J Bone Joint Surg Am. 2013;95(24):2170–6.
4. Wink MH, et al. Ultrasound imaging and contrast agents: a safe alternative to MRI? Minim Invasive Ther Allied Technol. 2006;15(2):93–100.
5. Greis C. Ultrasound contrast agents as markers of vascularity and microcirculation. Clin Hemorheol Microcirc. 2009;43(1–2):1–9.
6. Filipowska J, et al. The role of vasculature in bone development, regeneration and proper systemic functioning. Angiogenesis. 2017;20(3):291–302.
7. Giannoudis PV, et al. The diamond concept—open questions. Injury. 2008;39(Suppl 2):S5–8.
8. Molins IG, et al. Contrast-enhanced ultrasound in diagnosis and characterization of focal hepatic lesions. World J Radiol. 2010;2(12):455–62.
9. Greis C. Quantitative evaluation of microvascular blood flow by contrast-enhanced ultrasound (CEUS). Clin Hemorheol Microcirc. 2011;49(1–4):137–49.
10. Xu HX. Contrast-enhanced ultrasound: the evolving applications. World J Radiol. 2009;1(1):15–24.
11. Weber MA, Krix M, Delorme S. Quantitative evaluation of muscle perfusion with CEUS and with MR. Eur Radiol. 2007;17(10):2663–74.
12. D'Onofrio M, et al. Focal liver lesions: sinusoidal phase of CEUS. Abdom Imaging. 2006;31(5):529–36.
13. Fischer C, et al. Dynamic contrast-enhanced sonography and dynamic contrast-enhanced magnetic resonance imaging for pre-operative diagnosis of infected nonunions. J Ultrasound Med. 2016;35(5):933–42.
14. Krammer DS, Schmidmaier G, Weber MA, Doll J, Rehnitz C, Fischer C. Contrast-enhanced ultrasound (CEUS) quantifies the perfusion within tibial non-unions and predicts the outcome of revision surgery. Ultrasound Med Biol. 2018;44(8):1853–9.
15. Moghaddam A, et al. Treatment of atrophic tibia non-unions according to 'diamond concept': results of one- and two-step treatment. Injury. 2015;46(Suppl 4):S39–50.
16. Fischer C, et al. Dynamic contrast-enhanced magnetic resonance imaging (DCE-MRI) for the prediction of non-union consolidation. Injury. 2017;48(2):357–63.
17. Axelrad TW, Einhorn TA. Use of clinical assessment tools in the evaluation of fracture healing. Injury. 2011;42(3):301–5.
18. Claudon M, et al. Guidelines and good clinical practice recommendations for contrast enhanced ultrasound (CEUS) in the liver—update 2012: a WFUMB-EFSUMB initiative in cooperation with representatives of AFSUMB, AIUM, ASUM, FLAUS and ICUS. Ultraschall Med. 2013;34(1):11–29.
19. Piscaglia F, Bolondi L. The safety of Sonovue in abdominal applications: retrospective analysis of 23188 investigations. Ultrasound Med Biol. 2006;32(9):1369–75.

Stress Fractures

23

Christian Tesch

23.1 Synopsis

1.1 Rationale of application: X-ray-free direct representation of the connective tissue structures over a suspected fracture for the detection of direct or indirect signs of a stress fracture.

1.2 Level of evidence: III.

1.3 Indication: For the representation of the bone surface and the connective tissue structures above the bone if a stress fracture is suspected, especially if no diagnosis is possible on the X-ray image.

1.4 Age of the patient: Every age.

1.5 Contraindication: No.

1.6 Examination: Visualisation of the area suspected of fracture with high-resolution transducers (12–18 MHz), the transducer is placed at the point of greatest pain and always parallel to the axis of the bone. It is important to ensure that the cortical reflex is displayed most sharply. The transducer must be guided around the bone in parallel so that a suspected fracture cannot be overlooked if it is oblique. In addition to a cortical disruption, a periosteal thickening, lymphedema in the subcutaneous tissue and an inflammatory reaction in the power doppler are also to be found. If the cortical disruption is negative, the examination must be repeated after 7 days.

1.7 Indications for additional X-ray diagnostics: When detecting a stress fracture, a second imaging procedure should be used, preferably magnetic resonance imaging as the "golden standard" (Ammann et al. 2014) or X-ray to exclude other types of pathological fractures.

1.8 Pitfalls: Intraspongious stress fractures without an interruption of the cortex can be evidenced by ultrasound, here a change in the sound of the cortex with the extinction of the reverberation artifacts is to be sought (see Fig. 23.3).

1.9 Red flags: Pain in the femoral neck area with a suspected stress fracture should prompt be examined by magnetic resonance imaging because a dislocation is to be feared and ultrasound cannot reliably show the suspected fracture.

23.2 Introduction

Stress fractures have become very much in the focus of interest since the beginning of the sport and fitness movement because these often remain undetected and the athletes affected have to go to several places until the diagnosis is confirmed. The incidence in a meta-analysis is 3–6% for male athletes and military cadets and 9–10% for female athletes [1]. The lower extremity is disproportionately affected (95% of all stress fractures [2]), especially the metatarsal bones. The synonym "marching fracture" is derived from, because it can occur in soldiers after long marches, which was already described in the second half of the nineteenth century about fractures of the metatarsals in recruits [3].

Fractures of the metatarsalia 2–4 are to be described as uncritical fractures because the treatment even with weight-bearing has no risk of dislocation. Critical (or high-risk fractures ([1])) fractures are located on the calcar of the femur, the navicular, and the base of the MT5 because they need at least weight relief until bony consolidation. This explains that an early diagnosis is necessary to avoid the complication of a complete fracture, and thus, surgical treatment.

It is not easy to make a diagnosis because X-rays, the most widely used imaging method in orthopedic and trauma surgery practices, regularly fail in the early phase of this "disease" [4]. The symptoms often do not start suddenly, so a fracture is not considered. Because connective tissue reactions (swelling, reddening, diffuse pain) are particularly noticeable in the initial phase, the diagnosis of "inflammation" is made regularly, which is not fundamentally wrong but does not establish the connection to the injured bone.

C. Tesch (✉)
Praxis für Orthopädie und Chirurgie, Hamburg, Germany
e-mail: christian@gelenktesch.de

© Springer Nature Switzerland AG 2021
O. Ackermann (ed.), *Fracture Sonography*, https://doi.org/10.1007/978-3-030-63839-9_23

Ultrasound and magnetic resonance imaging are the imaging methods of choice for examining the connective tissue, whereby the latter is already generally considered the gold standard of diagnosis because of the complete imaging of the bone with cortical and cancellous parts [1, 5]. Ultrasound is assessed as too inconsistent in this meta-analysis [1]. This applies particularly to stress fractures of the sacrum, pelvis, and vertebrae, which are hardly accessible to ultrasound. However, since these are rare, but the fractures of the metatarsalia, the tibia, the fibula, the femur, and the humerus (in decreasing frequency) are significantly more common, ultrasound diagnosis is the imaging method of the first choice because the devices are widely used and the examination is basically simple. There is now good evidence of clear signs that confirm and rule out a fracture [6–11].

23.3 Development of a Stress Fracture

Stress fractures arise from a chronic overload of the bone, consisting of the compact cortex and the cancellous bone. Both structures can fracture separately or together, whereby the isolated cancellous bone fracture is not accessible for ultrasound diagnosis and is a domain of magnetic resonance imaging. Thus, in the further course, it is about the fractures of the cortex. Typically, this happens in the case of long bones.

If the pathogenesis of a stress fracture is accompanied by an underlying illness in addition to physical exertion (osteoporosis, rheumatoid arthritis, cortisone therapy, malnutrition, vitamin D deficiency), we call it "insufficiency fracture," because the bone is less resilient due to the comorbidity. At this point, the diagnosis of an insufficiency fracture needs further investigations for these pathologies. A distinction between stress and insufficiency fractures is not significant for diagnosis and therapy.

From technical reports on the material behavior of inorganic structures, we know the so-called vibration break (or "vibration break") is an example on crankshafts or connecting rods in engine construction. This leads to vibrations due to load changes, the energy of which is directly proportional to the vibration amplitude and frequency. When there are loads below the breaking limit, microcracks develop which can grow and lead to breakage when a critical size is reached. A fracture occurs under load change when the energy that acts on the material through bending, torsion, and shear exceeds the binding forces of the metal structure. Microcracks can be made visible in metal [12].

Transferred to the bones, fractures occur due to load changes, for example in the midfoot when walking, due to bending, torsion, and shear in the shaft of the metatarsal bones when they are footed and come up in opposite directions. The exact mechanism has not been researched with certainty, but work on shear forces on human bone suggests that they form microfractures essentially perpendicular to the osteons around them [11], thus following the lamellar structure of the bone. Bone has several properties that are important for understanding:

Cortical bone shows viscoelastic behavior, which means that its material properties depend on the rate of loading: when it is loaded faster, it is stiffer than when it is slow [13].

Cyclical loading (load change) leads to fatigue, but normal cortical bone can withstand up to one million load changes, which would correspond to a running distance of 1500 km.

Bone as a biological material is subject to constant remodeling processes so that "damage" is the drive power for repair processes. So-called microcracks [11, 13], which are mainly caused by shear, are constantly repaired and thus make up the "strong" bones. The RANKL system (Receptor Activator of NF-κB Ligand is a protein from the family of tumor necrosis factors) controls (the crack initiates the apoptosis of osteocytes that release the RANKL) the osteoclast absorption and thereby the osteoblastic bone cultivation [13].

In summary, the more the bone has been loaded, the more stable it is, which leads to interlamellar microfractures, which in turn activate and thus stabilize the new bone, "microcracks" only become a stress fracture in the clinical sense if the balance of the repair processes (attachment and disassembly) is disturbed and the bone metabolism is no longer able to heal the microcracks.

Especially for runners (medium and long distance) with the long-term load in almost the same walking distance on flat ground and very high training loads, the metatarsal bones, in particular, can quickly reach the limit of repairability. Training leads to the strengthening of the bone structures in the direction of the strength lines so that if the training intensity and frequency are selected wisely, the training-related strengthening of the bone structure leads the possible overload, and therefore, no fracture can occur. As described in detail above, stress and the bone remodeling processes are important in the regeneration phase leading to the strengthening of the bone structure (cortex and cancellous bone), which would then prevent breakage. This takes significantly longer than the adaptation of the cardiovascular system, muscles, tendons, and cartilage.

Imaging procedures should help to identify stress fractures at an early stage. This would be particularly helpful at the stage of development. For the reasons of intensive bone remodeling described above and the quasi need for "microcracks," it is pointless and also not possible to visualize this. But, and here ultrasound diagnostics should be mentioned first before major damage occurs, the representation of the first stages of a stress fracture would be particularly helpful.

23.4 Indication, Patients

If a stress fracture is suspected (pain in the forefoot, swelling, and reddening without previous injury, creeping course), ultrasound diagnostics is the simplest and safest non-radiation imaging. X-ray is always the second or third choice in this case! It is used in patients of all ages and genders, primarily athletes, because this clientele has by far the most common number of stress fractures.

23.4.1 Contraindication

Besides open wounds in the area under investigation, there are no contraindications.

23.5 Examination Technique and Course

23.5.1 Positioning

A special positioning is not necessary, the extremity to be examined should be comfortably held in position for the patient and easily accessible for the examiner.

23.5.2 Views

For long bones, a plane parallel to the longitudinal axis. For short bones, the view can be freely selected.

23.5.3 Setting

The "region of interest" is set centrally in the image and can be expanded by swiveling and moving around the extremity. For this purpose, the transducer is carefully placed on the point of maximum pressure pain and the bone is sonicated exactly orthogonally so that the cortical reflex is shown as sharply as possible (see Fig. 23.2).

23.5.4 Assessment, Diagnosis, Therapy

The basic principle of sonographic diagnostics is the detection of an interruption of the cortex (see Fig. 23.1) with linear transducers from 9 to 18 MHz always in the longitudinal course of the bone (applies to all long bones, with all other bones the axis is freely chosen). However, this gap in the cortex can be so minimal that it is beyond detection or a small fragment (such as a "bending wedge") can be found (see Fig. 23.2). There is always lymphedema (see Fig. 23.1), which is caused by inflammation, but the detection is nonspecific. In addition, the periosteum is examined for thickening or fluid accumulation (see Fig. 23.3). As a third sign, attention is paid to changes in the bone surface and the reverberation artifacts (see Figs. 23.4 and 23.5 and Table 23.2).

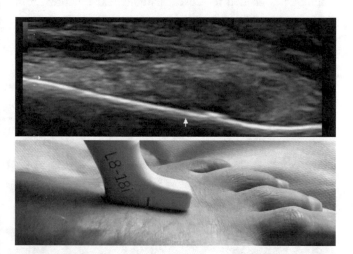

Fig. 23.2 18 MHz transducer placed on the point of maximum pain; Sonographic picture shows at the maximum pain point (SP) a small cortical interruption, a small fragment and with an extended low-echo zone above it as a sign of edema (From Tesch 2018b; Courtesy of Seminar-Label-Media)

Fig. 23.1 MT3 stress fracture (*) visible in the sonographic image with lymph floors (*white arrows*) and cortical bone, not visible in the X-ray (From Tesch 2018b; Courtesy of Seminar-Label-Media)

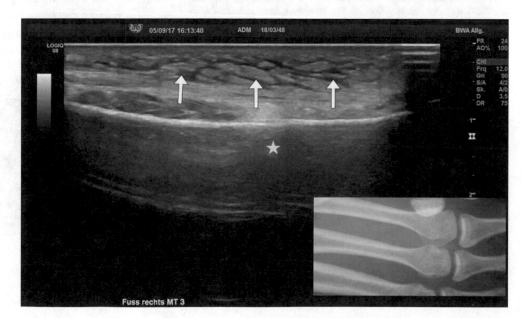

If the cortical interruption is missing, changes in the periosteum should be looked for. With a high-resolution transducer (16–18 MHz) the periosteum should be searched at the maximum pain point to determine whether it bulges out or appears thickened (see Fig. 23.3). Then a search is made for sound changes in the cortex and extinction of the reverberation artifacts. If this sign is also not found, the diagnosis is rather unlikely, but not excluded. This would be excluded if, 1 week after the first examination, all signs (cortical interruption, small fragment, periosteal lift or thickening, cortical thickening, or sound change with the extinction of the reverberation artifacts) cannot be detected.

With proof of the fracture line, the periosteal reaction, the cortex reaction, and changes in sound (reverberation artifacts), the diagnosis is assured. Important: another imaging technique is needed to prevent pathological fractures from being overlooked as a result of osteoporosis, tumors, or other pathologies.

X-ray diagnostics are generally suitable, if this has already taken place, then the second imaging is not necessary. As mentioned above, however, magnetic resonance imaging is the imaging of the first choice [14]. Here, the radiologist should definitely request a focused magnetic resonance imaging (max. 10 cm proximal and distal of the proven or suspected fracture), ideally in a side comparison. The imaging of the entire limb is unnecessary.

After the diagnosis of a stress fracture has been confirmed in the second imaging procedure, it must first be clarified whether the fracture is a high- or a low-risk fracture (see Table 23.1). In any case, the former is relieved in such a way that dislocation is reliably avoided. There are also reports that osteosynthesis is recommended, so that if a bilateral stress fracture of the cancellous bone and a fracture in a femoral neck are detected, a dynamic hip screw is implanted on both sides [15]. This explains that ultrasound diagnostics is the second choice to answer these questions.

The important question to clarify with ultrasound diagnostics is, to detect the time to increase the weight-bearing in fractures of low risk? This can be assessed well with the help of the fracture-healing stages [16, 17], see also chapter "Mechanical Monitoring of fracture healing with ultrasound" (Table 21.1).

23.6 Pitfalls and Red Flags

If symptoms persist after an initially normal examination, a second check should be carried out after a week so that a fracture is not overlooked.

In the case of proven fractures, underlying pathologies such as osteoporosis, bone mineralization disorders, and tumors should be excluded.

Intraspongious stress fractures with a cortical reaction without interruption can only be seen by erasing the reverberation artifacts (Figs. 23.6, 23.7, and 23.8).

Pain in the neck of the femur if a stress fracture is suspected must be clarified on the MRI in order to prevent a complete fracture under further stress. This pathology can be overlooked with the ultrasound.

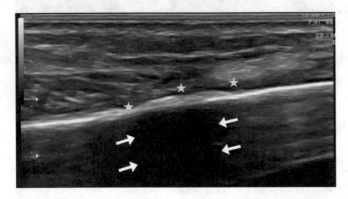

Fig. 23.3 15 MHz transducer placed dorsally on the painful area of the tibia, there cortex reaction with thickening (*), sound change with dorsal shadows and interruption of the reverberation artifacts (*white arrows*) (From Tesch 2018b; Courtesy of Seminar-Label-Media)

Fig. 23.4 12 MHz matrix transducer, panorama view, stress fracture of a tibia in a 15-year-old, at this time it was not clear to see. Symptoms started 7 days earlier. The only sign was the sound change with discreet darkening of the reverberation artifacts (*) (From Tesch 2018b; Courtesy of Seminar-Label-Media)

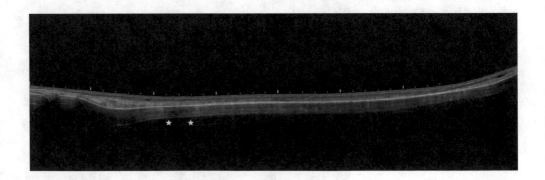

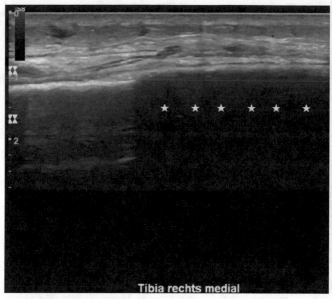

Fig. 23.5 12 MHz matrix transducer, 2 weeks after symptom onset. Stress fracture of the tibia, in a side comparison you can see the cortex–periosteal reaction with acoustic shadows and extinguishing the rever- beration artifacts (*), right part of the picture shows the healthy opposite side (From Tesch 2018b; Courtesy of Seminar-Label-Media)

Table 23.1 Risk that the fracture will dislocate and require additional measures

High risk	Low risk
Femoral neck, femoral	Fibula
Metatarsals 5	Metatarsals 2–4
Talus	Sacrum
Calcaneus	Cuneiformia
Radius, Ulna	

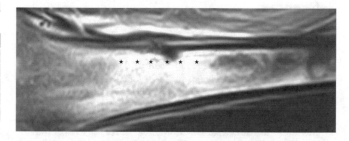

Fig. 23.6 Magnetic resonance imaging, eStir_longTE IR220 scythe, stress fracture 2 weeks after the onset of symptoms, the image shows the stress fracture at almost the same level as in Fig. 23.5, the cortical disruption was not seen sonographically (From Tesch 2018b; Courtesy of Seminar-Label-Media)

Table 23.2 Sound phenomena with a suspected stress fracture

Lymphedema (unspecific)
Cortical interruption
Small extra fragment
Thickening of the periosteum
Cortical reaction with thickening
Erase the reverberation artifacts

Fig. 23.7 12 MHz matrix transducer, stress fracture 8 weeks after the onset of symptoms, wide medial adjustment to the tibia, in something where the gap in the cortex was visible in Fig. 23.6, Powerdoppler sonography to demonstrate the intense inflammatory response during the healing process (From Tesch 2018b; Courtesy of Seminar-Label-Media)

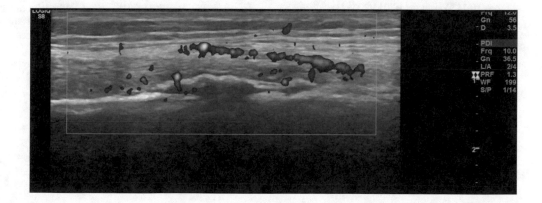

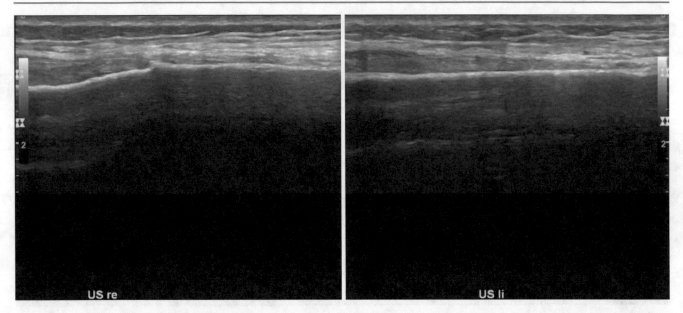

Fig. 23.8 12 MHz matrix transducer, tibia stress fracture, healing 3 months after the onset of symptoms, the healthy opposite side on the right. There is a small edge in the cortex, pay attention to the almost complete image of the reverberation artifacts on the right and left (see Table 23.2) (From Tesch 2018b; Courtesy of Seminar-Label-Media)

References

1. Wright AA, Hegedus EJ, Lenchik L, Kuhn KJ, Santiago L, Smoliga JM. Diagnostic accuracy of various imaging modalities for suspected lower extremity stress fractures: a systematic review with evidence-based recommendations for clinical practice. Am J Sports Med. 2016;44(1):255–63. doi:0363546515574066 [pii]. https://doi.org/10.1177/0363546515574066.
2. Liong SY, Whitehouse RW. Lower extremity and pelvic stress fractures in athletes. Br J Radiol. 2012;85(1016):1148–56. doi:85/1016/1148 [pii]. https://doi.org/10.1259/bjr/78510315.
3. Breithaupt MB. Zur Pathologie des menschlichen Fußes. Med Zeit. 1855;24:9.
4. Wolff R. Stressfraktur—Ermüdungsbruch—Stressreaktion. Dtsch Z Sportmed. 2001;52(4):5.
5. Mauch F, Kraus M, Gulke J, Ammann B. [MRI in musculoskeletal imaging: possibilities and limitations]. Unfallchirurg. 2014;117(3):227–234. https://doi.org/10.1007/s00113-013-2402-5.
6. Aksay E, Yesilaras M, Kilic TY, Tur FC, Sever M, Kaya A. Sensitivity and specificity of bedside ultrasonography in the diagnosis of fractures of the fifth metacarpal. Emerg Med J. 2015;32(3):221–5. doi:emermed-2013-202971 [pii]. https://doi.org/10.1136/emermed-2013-202971.
7. Duckham RL, Brooke-Wavell K, Summers GD, Cameron N, Peirce N. Stress fracture injury in female endurance athletes in the United Kingdom: a 12-month prospective study. Scand J Med Sci Sports. 2015;25(6):854–9. https://doi.org/10.1111/sms.12453.
8. Meardon SA, Willson JD, Gries SR, Kernozek TW, Derrick TR. Bone stress in runners with tibial stress fracture. Clin Biomech (Bristol, Avon). 2015;30(9):895–902. doi:S0268-0033(15)00209-0 [pii]. https://doi.org/10.1016/j.clinbiomech.2015.07.012.
9. Reinking MF, Austin TM, Bennett J, Hayes AM, Mitchell WA. Lower extremity overuse bone injury risk factors in collegiate athletes: a pilot study. Int J Sports Phys Ther. 2015;10(2):155–67.
10. Saglam F, Gulabi D, Baysal O, Bekler HI, Tasdemir Z, Elmali N. Chronic wrist pain in a goalkeeper; bilateral scaphoid stress fracture: a case report. Int J Surg Case Rep. 2015;7C:20–2. doi:S2210-2612(14)00460-X [pii]. https://doi.org/10.1016/j.ijscr.2014.12.025.
11. Tang T, Ebacher V, Cripton P, Guy P, McKay H, Wang R. Shear deformation and fracture of human cortical bone. Bone. 2015;71:25–35. doi:S8756-3282(14)00366-4 [pii]. https://doi.org/10.1016/j.bone.2014.10.001.
12. King A, Johnson G, Engelberg D, Ludwig W, Marrow J. Observations of intergranular stress corrosion cracking in a grain-mapped polycrystal. Science. 2008;321(5887):382–5. doi:321/5887/382 [pii]. https://doi.org/10.1126/science.1156211.
13. Kurth A, Lange U. Fachwissen Osteologie. München: Elsevier; 2018.
14. Ammann B, Mauch F, Schmitz B, Kraus M. [Weightings and sequences in magnetic resonance imaging in orthopedic surgery]. Unfallchirurg. 2014;117(3):197–198, 200–195. https://doi.org/10.1007/s00113-013-2399-9.
15. Khadabadi NA, Patil KS. Simultaneous bilateral femoral neck stress fracture in a young stone Mason. Case Rep Orthop. 2015;2015:306246. https://doi.org/10.1155/2015/306246.
16. Ricciardi L, Perissinotto A, Dabala M. External callus development on ultrasound and its mechanical correlation. Ital J Orthop Traumatol. 1992;18:223–9.
17. Ricciardi L, Perissinotto A, Dabala M. Mechanical monitoring of fracture healing using ultrasound imaging. Clin Orthop. 1993;293:71–6.

Part IV

Starting in Practice

Guide to Introduction to Everyday Clinical Practice

24

Ole Ackermann

The introduction of new methods into everyday clinical practice is always a challenge. Whether this is planned in a practice or clinic, the problems are similar. Colleagues who are used to X-ray findings must be convinced, dealing with new processes must be practiced and the diagnostic method itself trained. Complete, safe, and fast treatment of patients must also be guaranteed during the changeover phase.

Always have in mind: safety first! Whenever there is any doubt about the finding, an X-ray image is permitted and useful. Uncertainties always occur, especially in the initial phases, and it is best to eliminate them immediately and consistently. Nothing is more deadly for a new method than a misdiagnosis and many a hopeful start has failed because of it. Therefore, it is necessary to make the beginning safe for doctors and patients, with increasing routine the need for X-ray checks will be quickly minimized.

24.1 The Doctor Starts

To gain security as a beginner in sonographic fracture diagnostics, it is essential to first familiarize yourself with the possibilities and limits of the procedure. One has to realize that ultrasound always displays the surface of the bone. In the beginning, there are also often concerns that the examination could be painful. We can deny this from the experience of several thousand investigations.

The start of diagnostics with the distal fracture of the forearm is an ideal beginning. The fracture is often easy to visualize and, due to the high correction potential, very safe in therapy. In the beginning, it makes sense to carry out the sonographic examination, then commit yourself to a diagnosis and treatment, and then carry out an X-ray examination. The examiner will then see that the wrist SAFE leads to the goal. After 10–20 examinations, the necessary security is

usually available to use the X-ray examination only in exceptional cases.

Based on this basic knowledge, ultrasound diagnostics can then be extended to other areas.

Of course, a practical course to introduce the methodology is helpful.

24.2 Introduction to Practice

Experience has shown that the main obstacle is the availability of the (often the only) ultrasound device. The processes should be structured so that patients with suspected fractures are generally examined in the ultrasound room. Only then will the speed advantage of sonography become noticeable.

Even if the vast majority of parents prefer ultrasound imaging to X-ray diagnostics, it always happens that an X-ray examination is desired. In our experience, there is no point in discussing at this point, otherwise, the X-ray will be made up elsewhere. We proceed in such a way that we then carry out an ultrasound examination and also an X-ray image.

24.3 Introduction to the Clinic

If the clinic chief has not learned the method himself and wants to introduce it, there are several hurdles to be overcome. Every employee must be aware that the chief doctor is responsible for the clinic and, in case of doubt, is personally responsible for every procedure and every mistake. Therefore, he will only introduce a new method if he is convinced of its quality. To achieve this, it makes sense to first run ultrasound and X-ray diagnostics consistently in parallel and to present both in the X-ray discussion. Employees should also be free to use the technology in order to achieve good results.

If the method has proven its potential over time, a standard application can be discussed.

O. Ackermann (✉)
Department of Orthopedic Surgery, Ruhr-University Bochum, Bochum, Germany

© Springer Nature Switzerland AG 2021
O. Ackermann (ed.), *Fracture Sonography*, https://doi.org/10.1007/978-3-030-63839-9_24

Index

Printed in the United States
by Baker & Taylor Publisher Services